DON'T RAIN ON MY PARADE

Living a Full Life with Alzheimer's and Dementia

Richard Fenker, PhD

ISBN 978-0-9894600-1-9
First Printing, August 2016

Book design: n-kcreative.com
Printed in the United States of America

Published by: Cimarron International LLC
cimarroninternational.com
editor@cimarroninternational.com

For Mom, the ultimate care partner.

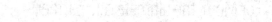

"Why not see us as a source of answers to our problems, rather than as a source of problems to which our caregivers need answers?"

—Richard Taylor
Alzheimer's from the Inside Out

CONTENTS

Living Life to Its Fullest

Embracing Technology to Add Quality to Your Life

Don't Rain on My Parade

Resources

FOREWORD

Social media and technology. Where would we be without them? At any given moment, you can have a conversation with someone 10,000 miles away, 10 minutes away, or within your own household. It puts you in contact with people who touch your life. It put me in touch with Richard Fenker.

Richard came to know me through our mutual contacts and from reading my blog. That's how he became aware of my life with early-onset Alzheimer's disease. Despite the fact that I have a disease that affects my brain, he still trusted me to write the foreword for his book. I was petrified at first, thinking to myself, "He's asking me, someone he has never met in person and someone with Alzheimer's disease, to write the foreword?" Then I thought, "Who better to write something about Alzheimer's than a person living *with* Alzheimer's?" My daily mantra, "I have Alzheimer's, *but* it doesn't have me!" kicked in, so I accepted.

My experience with Alzheimer's started in the same fashion as Richard's. We were both exposed to the disease in our teenage years through the lives of our grandfathers. I saw the physical effects it had on my mother and my aunt (my grandfather's care partners) and Richard saw the mental fear of his father, wondering if he would genetically inherit the disease. Thankfully, the gene passed him over. My mother wasn't as fortunate. She lived with Alzheimer's for over 10 years, passing away just three months after I was diagnosed. That will probably go down as one of the darkest times of my life. Seeing what it does to someone you love, someone who gave you life, is one thing ... knowing the same demise will happen to you is an entirely different experience. It was at that point I decided I was not going to let this disease define me.

Richard Fenker's book speaks to everyone living with dementia. You see, Alzheimer's really doesn't have me. I don't like when people say I suffer from Alzheimer's or I'm an Alzheimer's patient. I'm simply "living with Alzheimer's" and, although each day is a challenge, I live it fully. I'm still here—thinking, feeling, understanding, loving—and if I look a little different to you from the outside, on the inside, I'm the same person. I'm Brian, the same Brian as before, just living with a disease. For the first time an author, from the outside, has attempted to enter my world to join me on my journey.

Richard immersed himself in the lives of people who have (had) Alzheimer's—individuals like the late Richard Taylor, John Sandblom, and yours truly, just to name a few, by reading their books and blogs, having conversations with them, and trying to understand what these individuals did to make their lives as positive as possible. It took courage and empathy on his part to find out not just what it was like to have the disease but what it was like to *live with* the disease.

He read about the problems and issues we had and figured out what he could do to help, using technology, sharing supportive advice with care partners, and using any other information vehicle he came across. Thankfully, he left no stone unturned, but I have a feeling he will soon be searching for more stones to turn over.

The magic of Fenker's book is that it is all about me and people like me. Everyone living with Alzheimer's has to make a crucial choice—whether or not to show up the next day and decide to live fully. When you make this choice, it opens a whole world of possibilities for you that offer joy, humor, the gift of communication, hope, and much more. This is not a book written to my care partners, physicians, and others watching from the sidelines. It's for me.

Alzheimer's disease is not like cancer, heart disease, HIV/AIDS, or any other disease that has preventive measures. Alzheimer's has none. Sadly, Alzheimer's has no survivors. No longer is this a disease of the elderly. Individuals in their 30s, 40s, and 50s are now being diagnosed with early-onset Alzheimer's disease. These are young people with families and their whole lives before them. Time becomes very limited. It then becomes a choice as to whether you want to live it positively or not. As I said, I chose the positive route.

Fenker is a technologist and inventor. While the modern world has moved on with iPhones and other mobile devices that attach to thousands of apps that stretch the imagination with possibilities, he offers MindPartner (using a companion mind that stores my personal history and then delivers it back to me when needed). It suggests a way to expand the potential of my world and bring me many varieties of practical help.

If you are living with dementia today, you know that your life is a battleground, as you struggle to maintain your independence and your integrity as a person in a world that is often negative and not always understanding. I think this book gets inside that world and can empower you, and your care partners, with the tools to "live a full life."

Don't Rain on My Parade: Living a Full Life with Alzheimer's and Dementia takes you on a journey, starting with making choices about how you will live your life, ending with embracing death, and traveling along all points in between. Yes, just as death is a part of everyday life, death is also a part of the Alzheimer's life. The difference is how it comes to be.

Richard does a phenomenal job not only as an author but also as a guide through the world of Alzheimer's, taking us on this strange and wonderful journey.

—Brian LeBlanc

Author of blog, *Alzheimer's: The Journey*

PREFACE

My introduction to Alzheimer's disease and dementia comes from experiences with family members. My grandfather, Fodda, was diagnosed with Alzheimer's at age 88 and lived another eight years, most of these in a nearby traditional nursing home. This experience was so ugly that my dad planned his later years to be sure that he did not have to repeat this scenario. Fodda's daughter, my aunt Emilou, was diagnosed with Alzheimer's at age 90 and lived another 12 years. Her last years were spent in a warm, professional setting, with a home-like atmosphere and a special memory-care unit—with a daughter and grandchildren nearby.

I have a PhD in psychology and I am a professor emeritus at TCU in Fort Worth, where I taught for many years; one of my specialties was the study of human consciousness. From my limited exposure to both Fodda and Emilou, it seemed to me that a great deal was happening within their minds that we didn't understand. They were both frustrated for a long period as their verbal skills and general ability to function in the world were diminished, but a good part of this frustration was tied to their caregivers and problems with communication.

A lot was happening in their minds that they could not say or communicate.

My first book on this topic, *The Long Moment: Giving a Voice to the Alzheimer's Mind,* describes some of what happens to consciousness as the disease progresses, and how people with dementia and their caregivers can do a better job of communicating. One of the products that came from the book, now being used today in a variety of settings, was the Alzheimer's Communication Cards. These are simple tools to help someone with limited verbal skills "speak" what is on their mind with text and images.

As I continued to learn more about what it was like to live with dementia from working with caregivers, one thing jumped out at me. People typically live years in the early and middle stages of the disease and, during this period, are very conscious of the world around them and normal in many respects—even though they may not be functioning well in our shared Earth-reality. We harm these individuals with our negative doom-and-gloom approach to Alzheimer's and the stigma that we assign to them. We diminish their personhood with our tendency to treat them as children. What if, instead of scaring people, we focused on bringing as much quality as possible to their lives by adding "long moments" that are joyful, active, entertaining, or just normal? How would we do this?

The answer to this question has many components, represented by the chapters in this book. All are focused on helping you live your life with dementia as completely and joyfully as possible. Several chapters deal with the role that technology can play in helping, based on another part of my history as an inventor and founder of several Internet companies. We normally think of today's technology as something designed for teenagers, businesspeople, or a generation of iPhone users—not the elderly, especially those with dementia. *But what if we took the best that current technology has to offer and used it to improve the quality of life for individuals with Alzheimer's/dementia?* What would that be like?

It is my belief that it could make a huge difference, one measured by thousands of positive moments added to the life of each person living with Alzheimer's today, including you. We don't need to wait for the right kind of treatment or drug to fix the disease. Right now, in a short time, with smart use of technology already developed and a change in attitude, we have much to offer you.

This book and the associated program called MindPartner (based on the idea of saving your memories and personal history in a companion mind and then feeding it back to you over time as needed) is the result. I offer them both with love and respect for you, if you are diagnosed with Alzheimer's or any other form of dementia, and for your family of care partners. (While the book is for anyone with dementia, I use the words Alzheimer's and dementia interchangeably throughout because Alzheimer's is the most common and most familiar version.)

I write these words with humility. I am not a dementia professional, nor a caregiver for a family member with dementia, but rather an inventor with an idea I think can help. Throughout this book, I will be speaking to you, the individual with dementia, as if I could somehow enter your mind in its current state, know what you are experiencing, and give you advice.

Obviously, this is not possible; I cannot penetrate your reality any more that you can enter mine. Instead, I am limited to combining the stories and wisdom from people living with Alzheimer's, scientific information, and the experiences of caregivers and dementia professionals, plus a healthy dose of my own intuition. I will be speaking directly to *you* but with this collective voice. Please forgive me when my general statements miss the heart of your unique and personal life with dementia. There are few generalities here; I recognize that you are alone on a very individual journey and at best my words can, at times, overlap with your reality.

—Richard Fenker

CARE PARTNER RULES OF THE ROAD
(How I Expect You to Treat Me)

1. **Please become my best friend and advocate**—and relinquish your former role as my spouse, child, grandchild, other relative, or friend. It is much more helpful to support who I am now than to hang onto who I used to be—and as a best friend, you can do this.

2. **Always relate to me as the complete, adult person whom you know** me to be inside, regardless of what I say or do on the outside. I am still me inside and will always be that me that you know.

3. **Please learn to listen beyond the words that you hear me speak** and focus on the message that I am trying to communicate. Taking my words too literally will often miss what I am attempting to share.

4. **Please understand that my silence and tendency to withdraw often just reflect my fear of making mistakes.** Your unconditional acceptance of me, at any moment, without evaluation or judgment is essential to my well-being and my willingness to speak out.

5. **Please learn to "come to me" in any situation where we are communicating or I need your help.** Attempts to test me or pull me back into your reality won't work and will only frustrate us both. Each day, my journey may take me further from our shared world. I cannot return, so you must join me wherever I am, in the moment.

6. **My frustration and anger are a normal part of the battle I fight each day,** with myself and with the world, to remain competent, communicate my needs, and live a full life. They are not a judgment of you. I will not always be quiet, polite, and logical. So be it. Your understanding and patience with me make it possible to move past these moments.

7. **Please don't be concerned with the repetitive pattern behavior that you may see as my short-term memory skills decline.** I know it may frighten, confuse, and frustrate you. Please don't be concerned. Inside my mind, I will not be aware of the repetitions—and you are serving me best just by joining me again in the moment, even if that moment has happened many times.

8. **Please respect my reality!** My experiences at any moment, while they may be bizarre to you, are very real to me.

9. **Please slow down and be patient with me.** There is no hurry. My thinking and speaking take more time, so don't rush to fill in missing words or complete a task when I act confused. Every bit of independence you encourage by not rushing in is a gulp of fresh air to my confidence and well-being.

10. **Laugh with me and entertain me with humor.** Look my disability straight in the eye and deal with me directly, as an adult, with a smile on your face. I welcome the opportunity for laughter and a lightness of being.

"While I have the facility to do so, I want to communicate to others, to those who will face this demon some day and those who love them, that with the proper medical direction, life strategies, faith, and humor, one can prevail in the moment and lead a productive life for as long as possible."

—Greg O'Brien,
On Pluto: Inside the Mind of Alzheimer's

BEGINNING YOUR LIFE WITH DEMENTIA

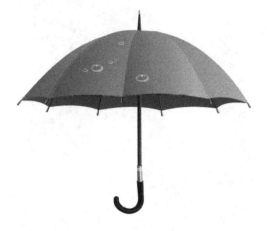

1

Making a Choice

Once I accepted my diagnosis of early-onset Alzheimer's, I decided to meet it the way I have met all difficulty in my life—with a spit-in-your-eye attitude and a sense of humor.

So I unofficially adopted the Cheshire Cat as my mascot. "'All right,' said the Cat; and this time it vanished quite slowly, beginning with the end of the tail, and the grin, which remained some time after the rest of it had gone."

So that's my philosophy: All right, Alzheimer's got me, but I plan on vanishing slowly and having my grin remain for a long time.

—Donnamarie Baker, blog member,
www.facebook.com/pages/Memory-People

This is a short guide for you, if you are in the early stages of Alzheimer's (or other forms of dementia), and for your caregivers. It's a book about how you live the rest of your life. The choices you make will guide that life in directions that are positive and fulfilling or negative and limited. I know, with an Alzheimer's diagnosis, it may not be obvious that you have a choice, but you do. You may not be able to take a pill or have surgery to produce a cure, but you can choose to influence the quality of your life while living with the disease. You can choose to live life to its fullest, completely and joyfully.

Part of the reason you may not recognize that you have a choice is that the primary voice of the Alzheimer's community in the United States, the Alzheimer's Association, lacks choices for individuals with Alzheimer's. The association's focus is on finding a cure or a helpful intervention and supporting organizations with this goal, not on insuring the quality of your life with dementia. It is an ally for you but not your organization; it serves physicians, researchers, fundraisers, administrators, educators, and caregivers. This is safe territory because all of these groups understand goals and mission statements, and benefit from the solutions offered.

The "Black Hole" of Dementia

Your landscape as a person living with dementia is vastly different. Your world is the Wild West, the Amazon jungle, and Antarctica all rolled up into a new planet that I call Altzair. Our fear of Alzheimer's has blocked us from exploring and understanding this planet. Unlike cancer, where the concept of cancer survivor has generated a culture of love, funding, and support, there are no Alzheimer's survivors, and tales of people living on this new planet and doing well are difficult to find. It's similar to a black hole; once you enter the gravity field of dementia, much of your light and experience is trapped and can no longer escape. The Alzheimer's community complicates this issue by remaining bogged down in the fear and hardships that the disease presents. Instead of bracelets celebrating victory over cancer, you have to live with "The Longest Day," "The Long Goodbye," and other negative concepts that claim to represent your voice.

A common perspective within this community is that the Alzheimer's diagnosis begins a grieving process for you and your caregivers that will last the rest of your life. While it comes as no surprise that you and your caregivers are grieving the loss of the pre-dementia life you were planning, and will certainly miss this life in the future, is grief all that is left for you? If you have just received the diagnosis, it can be like a punch in the stomach that takes your breath away and you may need to grieve for some time. But this isn't a lifelong process unless you decide to make it one.

Choosing to Live a Full Life

Why would you want to give up the potential for a full life in order to continue grieving? Thousands of people each year take another path based on a different choice, the choice to grieve for the moment and then gradually let go of the grief, accept the fact that you have dementia, and, with a smile on your face, decide to continue living as completely and happily as possible. There is no question that you will be challenged on this path; however, there is also no doubt that choosing to release your grief, accept your present circumstances, and move on with a positive outlook will have a great deal to do with your future happiness.

Atul Gawande frames this choice very clearly in his excellent book, *Being Mortal: Medicine and What Matters in the End*. At any moment in time, our consciousness is filled with hopes and fears. You can probably see these operating in your own mind. Typically, when we are happy and living life to its fullest our hopes dominate our fears, so that the content of our consciousness is mostly positive and focused on good outcomes. When our fears dominate our consciousness, however, we increase the chance for negative outcomes to occur and make positive emotions such as happiness or joy more difficult to find. A fearful outlook also increases our stress levels and erodes our physical well-being. We get what we expect—and expecting negative results facilitates their occurrence.

A dementia/Alzheimer's diagnosis in today's world gives the fearful part of your consciousness a huge shot of adrenalin for many reasons, since fear is often used as the basis for fundraising. You are fortunate if your physician did not feed into this negativity based on the absence of a medical solution or preventive measures. This simple scale illustrates what happens to many people after the diagnosis, as the fearful parts of consciousness become dominant.

Living with Alzheimer's isn't like knocking your head against a brick wall and suddenly entering a coma, where you lose all awareness. For most people, the early/moderate stages of the disease, where you retain your identity and consciousness, will last many years. My perspective and the message of this book is that, with a little help, you can add thousands of moments of normal living and joy to your life during this period.

Person-centered Care

Taking a positive approach to Alzheimer's is not a new idea within the dementia community. Person-centered care, with its focus on improving the subjective experience of the individual rather than on implementing a medical or facility-based regimen, was introduced in the 1990s and is used in many settings today. What may be new for you and your caregivers, however, is the simple idea that adopting a negative approach to dementia is not helpful, because it blocks your opportunity to live a rich, full life.

Richard Taylor, one of the giants of the Alzheimer's world, who died in 2015, was still speaking publicly on dementia 10 years after the diagnosis. Here is part of his blog post from May 22, 2014:

"We all experience life differently . . . We all interpret our experiences differently. But we are similar in both our experiences and interpretations. Where we are different is in what we do with these."

Your future with Alzheimer's is not a given. You may or may not be like Richard and others, writing blogs for many years; but, regardless of what is happening inside your consciousness, you will still be you. What I want you to do now is make a simple choice: the choice to continue to march in the parade that is your life for as long as possible, living for moments of joy and peace and contentment, and living as a complete, independent, adult being. I want you to face the negative winds swirling around you, face them head on and move forward, ready to do battle, with a grin on your face and a glint in your eye.

Are you still in doubt? Here is a brief story that reminds us how strong our beliefs can be in shaping the outcomes in our lives:

A great Japanese warrior named Nobunaga decided to attack the enemy although he had only 1/10 the number of men the opposition commanded. He knew that he would win, but his soldiers were in doubt.

On the way, he stopped at a Shinto shrine and told his men, "After I visit the shrine, I will toss a coin. If heads comes up, we will win; if tails, we will lose. Destiny holds us in her hand."

Nobunaga entered the shrine and offered a silent prayer. He came forth and tossed a coin. Heads appeared. His soldiers were so eager to fight that they won their battle easily.

"No one can change the hand of destiny," his attendant told him after the battle.

"Indeed not," said Nobunaga, showing a coin that had been doubled, with heads facing either way.

In truth, both sides of your coin speak to living fully and joyfully, because in facing the conundrum that Alzheimer's presents, you are already embracing the opportunity to continue your parade. You know that this decision will test you, but you accept this as you prepare for the journey ahead. You may also face a number of limitations and challenges that will demand preparation and help from others. As you make your choice, you understand that much of the joy and normality in your life will depend on these companions or caregivers and their support.

Perhaps you're thinking, "OK. I'll make the choice to live a full life with dementia. I want to explore that option. That's the easy part. But what comes next? How do I accomplish this? How do I need to behave to make this happen?" While the remaining chapters in this book offer lots of suggestions to guide you, your journey needs to begin somewhere—and that beginning depends on your compass. It needs to be pointed at all times in the direction of True North, toward joy and happiness, to receive the most favorable winds.

Finding Happiness

Choosing to live fully and joyfully with dementia means choosing moment by moment to be happy. From now on, you will be doing your best to bring happiness into your life by choosing to interpret what happens in your world in a way that will make you happy. To a large degree, you create the world and what you feel and experience with the conversations that take place in your mind. Some of these conversations may be negative. In a later chapter, I describe the importance of letting go of any conflicts that can destroy happiness by replacing it with anxiety and frustration.

The choice you are making now to live life to its fullest begins with the decision to find happiness whenever and wherever possible on your journey. The next chapter covers this topic in more detail as I describe the simple but profound results of current research on aging and happiness.

The Daily Battle

Now for the bad news. I would like to say that making these choices will be easy, but unfortunately, that may not be the case. There is always a challenging side to any decision and the negatives associated with Alzheimer's can be strong, pervasive, and unconsciously supported by caregivers and others who mean well. To keep your bearings and your compass headed north in the midst of dementia's swirling winds, you may need to do battle every day. You will need to pay attention to two principal foes. One you already know well; it is the part of you that wants to discourage you, frustrate you, and pull you into a negative outlook on today and the future. This book is full of tools and ideas to help here.

The other foe is less obvious at times because it comes disguised as an ally, offering help while at the same time marginalizing you. This is the community of family, caregivers, physicians, and others around you who, for a variety of reasons, don't get the concept that you are a complete, independent human being— not a child, an emotional cripple, or the subject of a fundraising campaign on the horrors of dementia. Both of these foes can potentially assault you daily and pull you down unless you put up a good fight, which you can do.

This is not surprising. No one who breaks a leg, has radiation treatment for cancer, undergoes surgery to remove or repair an organ, or experiences any of a thousand other health problems or cures, does so without some inconvenience. Dementia is inconvenient. You can count on being inconvenienced; but, as Greg O'Brien reminds us in his book *On Pluto: Inside the Mind of Alzheimer's*, there is no shortage of good mentors here: Glen Campbell, who continued to perform for years after the onset of the disease (beautifully described in the documentary "I'll Be Me"); Pat Summitt, former coach of the Tennessee women's basketball team; Richard Taylor, the teacher and writer I quote throughout this book; Greg himself; and many others. As Greg says, "And so it is with chronic illness, good days and bad days. You get knocked down, you get back up. Again and again. You find a way to win."

Unlike many others who are ill, you still have a lot of life to live. I hope you choose to live it to its fullest and do so joyfully.

Living with Hope: Choosing Not to Have Alzheimer's

I've saved the best for last. To end this chapter, let's go back to the time when you were noticing some symptoms of dementia but had not received an Alzheimer's diagnosis. Then you were part of a large population who have the disease but don't know it. Why does this matter?

What if it were possible to live your life with Alzheimer's and have this life be so normal that neither you nor those around you could detect the presence of the disease! Is this a fantasy? Could it ever be possible to live with Alzheimer's and live somewhat normally? Surprisingly, the answer is "yes." As you will see later, many thousands of people each year live full lives with Alzheimer's, lives that are so normal the disease is not diagnosed until after their deaths! Is it possible for you to be part of this population? Probably not, since you are already showing dementia symptoms; however, the choices you make in this chapter and the next give your sails a big push in the right direction. Is it possible for you to learn some things from this population that can help you? Absolutely. Lifestyle, attitude, and other factors, including an important neurological concept called cognitive reserve, play a significant role.

The purpose of this book is to support your positive choice to continue with the parade by offering the ideas, plans, and tools you will need to live a complete and joyful life—and to find happiness in as many moments as possible.

KEY POINTS

- An Alzheimer's diagnosis forces you to take a deep breath, spend the time you need to grieve, and then, when you are ready, make a choice.

- You can choose to buy into the negativity and fearfulness of the current Alzheimer's community, or you can choose to continue to live your life as fully, as positively, and as independently as possible as an adult being.

- A large community of people and organizations is waiting to support you when you choose to continue living a full life.

- There are no limits on what is possible for you. Despite living with dementia, you will still choose and create much of the reality that you experience. Your choice now can send your world in a positive direction.

- Living positively with dementia is not an easy choice. It will challenge you every day. But once you make this choice, it will add many thousands of quality moments to your life and to the lives of your care partners.

Ideas for your life? How might you act on them? What is the first step?

2

Focus on Happiness

One can choose to crawl up on the couch and feel sorry for themselves, watch this disease take from them little by little. Or they can focus on what they still have. What they still can do.

People say I am courageous for what I am doing. Posting or talking about my journey. It's not that. It's not even close. I am merely doing what many others do, talking about my journey, and I am telling about the journey of those who no longer can communicate.

I tell everyone who asks me, "How are you?" I tell them I am thankful. Because I am. I could be worse. I will be worse. I am indeed thankful that I have my wife, our family and most important my God to talk to.

I am a thankful man, doing the best I can do, "While I Still Can . . ."
—Rick Phelps, *Memory People Blog*

Happiness is the most personal of concepts, yet we often associate it with external things—wealth, beauty, lifestyle, and physical comfort would be common examples. Research shows that when we evaluate the lifestyles of others, we expect wealthy people or intelligent people to be happier, even though we recognize that is often not the case. While there may be some association among these external factors, especially health and personal happiness, in general, the concept of happiness, like most other emotions and feelings (such as feeling stressed) depends largely on internal factors, on what is happening in our minds as we experience the world.

In Chapter 1, I described happiness as one of the essential choices you must make to live life fully with dementia. In this chapter, I will share more detail on the the importance of this choice and how to live happily regardless of whether, at the moment, you consider yourself a happy person.

Research on Aging and Happiness

To begin, let's examine some recent research on aging and happiness, and the surprising conclusions that resulted. We all know special people who, as they age and deal with the inconveniences that aging brings, manage to keep a positive, happy attitude. They bounce back quickly from physical problems, changes in their environment, the death of close family or friends, and almost everything else the world can throw at them.

The National Science Foundation (NSF) Institute on Aging followed a group of 10,000 people age 70 and older for a period of 10 years, using a semi-annual survey to measure health, happiness, and many other factors. What they learned surprised them, because it occurred over and over, regardless of the age of the individual when the study started, their residence (home or residential care facility), and the medical conditions they were dealing with.

What did they find? People who perceived themselves as happy received the following nice rewards:

- They lived longer (by 4.3 years on average).

- They lived happier (62 percent of their experiences were judged to be positive, compared to 34 percent for the rest of the population).

- They lived healthier, based on the medical assessment tool used in the study.

- They attracted more social support from family and caregivers.

As you can see, being happy regardless of the circumstances can add a number of positive benefits. While this research wasn't focused on a population with dementia (although some in the sample did have dementia), the broad and consistent nature of these results means that their findings most likely apply to you and others with Alzheimer's. Being happy supports your choice to live life to its fullest.

But perhaps you're thinking, how do you do this if happiness is based on internal, not external, factors? How do you change the programs that are already part of your personality that might be making you happy or unhappy? To answer this question, let me describe a simple exercise that I did for many years with students in my class on human consciousness.

A Happiness Experiment

Each day for two weeks, the students were asked to observe the things that made them happy during the day and then to list them in a notebook before they went to bed. Most students experienced two similar results. First, during the two-week period, the lists of happy experiences each day grew longer. Looking for happy experiences led to finding or creating more of them. Second, at the end of the exercise, the students rated their own level of happiness as being higher than when they started. In other words, a simple change in behavior quickly affected how the students were feeling. Surprisingly, a few students in each class would drop out of the exercise early—typically because the heightened experience of happiness was considered to be sinful and inappropriate.

Similar results have been observed for many different populations in many different settings. Focusing on things that make you happy makes you happier. Such a focus affects your mind in two ways: First, it tunes parts of your mind to seek out happy experiences; second, it helps you avoid giving a negative spin to an event that could have been interpreted positively or neutrally.

Choices that Support Happiness: Don't Sweat the Small Stuff

The NSF research on aging was very clear on this point. People who judged themselves to be happy and experienced this feeling most of the time were also people who had learned not to get upset over small things that didn't work out as well as they expected. They learned to ignore these things, or reinterpret them. Let's face it, life is full of small things that can annoy or stress you—if you let them. Learning to let go of these things, to ignore them or react to them in a neutral manner, is a big part of staying happy.

Your life with Alzheimer's can be filled with inconvenient things you could choose to be upset about—your memory doesn't work properly, people don't understand you, and daily habits can be a chore. Part of this is dementia, while another part is simply due to normal aging. How are you going to react to these kinds of situations in the future? You are not! Whenever possible you will simply acknowledge them, accept them, let them go, and move on to other thoughts or actions that are neutral or positive and associated with happiness.

Consider, for example, a person you deal with regularly that you find annoying. Wait a minute! Who put you on a pedestal that allows you to be the person who can be annoyed and to judge which others become annoying persons? The same logic can be applied to most anything: meals, personal needs, TV shows, nursing care. You can take the time to judge all of these and find plenty not to like if this is your choice—or you can choose to let them go and focus on what makes you happy. You can let go of things or people that annoy you by reinterpreting them.

The Power of a Happiness Checklist

The exercise I used with the class is a good one for you, especially with the help of a partner to monitor it. Make a Happiness Checklist—a list of everything you can think of that makes you happy, and when you discover something new, add it to the list. At dinner time or before bed, sit down with a spouse or friend or caregiver and go over the list, noting the things you did that day that added happy moments.

This is all you need to do. As simple as this exercise sounds, when done regularly, it has enormous power to cut through the fog of dementia and add many positive moments to your life.

Happiness also Has Physical Benefits

Every disease has mental and physical components. Hundreds of books and thousands of research studies document the role that a healthy mental attitude plays in illness. Put simply, there are physical changes associated with any illness, but the manifestation of these changes in our consciousness and every-day experience varies a great deal depending on our attitude.

A positive outlook on life, based in part on our personal happiness, helps to keep illness at bay by enhancing our defenses. It also gives us a way to interpret the experience of any disorder more as an inconvenience than as something that makes us "sick."

Chart 2A shows a simple curve that describes the overall quality of life (a combination of physical and mental health) a typical person might expect in the last 10 years of life. Because it is an idealized curve, it doesn't show the bumps that would send it higher or lower for brief periods. Rather, it just illustrates a gradual decline over time. Many people without a major disease or life-ending illness will experience a gradual decline similar to this.

Chart 2A

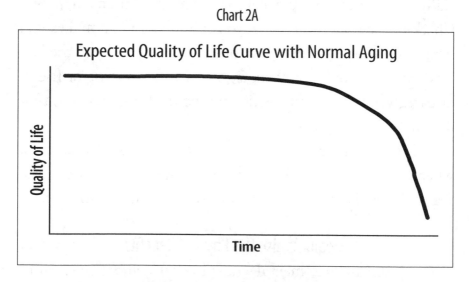

An Alzheimer's diagnosis can dramatically change the shape of this curve, depending on what choice you make. In Chart 2B, you will notice two lines, the black line identical to the one from

Chart 2B

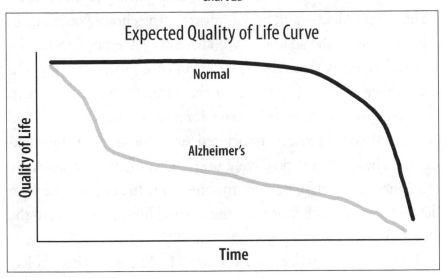

the previous chart and a second gray line with a steep drop early followed by a long, gradual decline.

The bottom line illustrates what our current negative approach to dementia can do to our expectations about life quality. Here you can see that the diagnosis brings an immediate and steep decline to the curve, based on our perceived ideas of what to expect. This lower line reflects the full weight of society's attitudes toward Alzheimer's and the absence of a cure. For many families, anticipation of what will happen to the quality of life after the diagnosis is like falling off a cliff. It is sudden and dramatic. To say this represents a negative view of Alzheimer's is an understatement, but I recognize that it may also reflect how you are viewing your life at this moment.

Avoid the Bus

There is no doubt that, over time, dementia will affect your quality of life; but there is also no reason for you to be "thrown under the bus" by your recent diagnosis. Now you can understand the problem—and how important the choice you made in Chapter 1 is to the solution. We currently have no cure for the physical changes that Alzheimer's will cause in your body and mind. That is just a fact that, for the moment, we must accept. However, we do have help now for the negative mental and emotional consequences associated with the disease. By making the choice to live positively and find happiness in as many moments as possible, you are making your life experience with dementia look much more like the normal life-quality line in the above charts.

This choice is under your control. To live with this choice, you will need some help from caregivers and technology, but this help is available to you now. Focusing on the things that bring happiness to your life, moment by moment, is the magic potion. It works by helping you to "cure" much of the psychological pain associated with the disease, by replacing negative thoughts with positive ones and by focusing on living as well and completely as possible.

The Problem of Depression

Is depression complicating your experience of living with dementia? If so, it adds to the challenge of finding happiness. The thoughts and feelings associated with depression often anchor the negative end of the happiness scale. If you are experiencing these kinds of symptoms, it is essential to replace them with something more positive.

Living with dementia in the early stages can challenge, as you already know, how you feel about yourself. It forces you to rewrite some of the rules of everyday living, your social relation-ships, your plans for the future, and much more. At the heart of these changes are the broad issues of competency and control. Not only can you see and feel the consequences of not func-tioning as well now as in your previous adult life, but you can imagine a future where these challenges only increase over time. For many living with Alzheimer's or any form of dementia, this can lead to depression.

Brian LeBlanc, living with early-onset Alzheimer's, describes his challenges:

. . . most people who suffer from depression wear a mask every day, but no one else sees it. It's the face they want you to see. It's the face they need to put on in order to face the world each and every day. At times, depending upon the situation, the mask will come off. Other times, the mask stays on because it can't be removed. That's when some people start thinking dark thoughts.

If you know someone who is suffering from depression, reach out to them, but realize, you can't fix them. The best thing you can do is "be there" for them. If they need or want to talk, let them. Don't insert your thoughts or advice, "just listen." If they want to just sit in silence with you, "let them." Don't continually ask them, "what's wrong?" "Are you OK." If they need to cry, "hold them," give them comfort and let them release. If it goes beyond that, you may want to suggest that they seek professional help.

Depression and dementia go hand in hand, especially in the early stages. Not everyone with dementia is depressed, but depression is a common response to the changes in life that accompany a diagnosis. To make this issue even more complicated, the symptoms of depression and dementia can be very similar. Things such as loss of interest in favorite activities, reduced concentration, social withdrawal, and memory problems are shared in both cases. What is important here is recognizing whether depression is a problem, because the treatment is not the same as for dementia.

Are you dealing now with depression in addition to dementia? How can you tell, since dementia alone may have similar symptoms? You probably already know the answer to these questions. At the core of depression is your mood and how you feel about things. Do you feel sad, hopeless, and discouraged most of the time? Are you finding that visits from family and friends bring little pleasure? Are activities that you once enjoyed no longer enjoyable? In reading the first chapter, Making a Choice, was your response negative? Did you think, "It doesn't matter. No option now is a good one." If you're experiencing several of these feelings, there is a good chance that you're depressed.

Managing Depression and Dementia

How do you deal with depression and dementia at the same time? First, I encourage you and your caregivers to go online and find some of the excellent materials on this topic published by the Alzheimer's Association, the Mayo Clinic, the Alzheimer's Society, and others. Understanding the symptoms of depression and your responses to them is a great first step toward reducing its impact. These organizations offer many ideas and tools that can help.

I would caution you not use antidepressants without the advice of your physician. Research suggests that past-generation drugs, such as tricyclic antidepressants, are likely to have undesirable side effects for you. Using any mood-altering drugs can complicate your goal to live fully and independently.

Despite this caution, a newer class of antidepressants called SSRIs (for selective serotonin reuptake inhibitors) that affect serotonin levels in the brain offer some promise and are the first choice of many physicians. They are effective in treating many types of depression with minimal side effects and, as a bonus, current research suggests they may prevent or delay the onset of Alzheimer's by driving down the production of beta-amyloid proteins. If confirmed, this could be a ground-breaking finding for the dementia community, but this is still a very new idea and more testing is needed. I recommend that if you are dealing with depression, you discuss this option with your physicians.

Some non-drug approaches to depression offered by the Alzheimer's Association include:

- Support groups or individual counseling

- A predictable routine or daily schedule

- A happiness checklist

- Celebrating small successes

- Encouraging others to use active listening to acknowledge your feelings and needs

- Nurturing with favorite foods, emotional support, and inspirational activities

- Finding ways to reassure yourself that you will not be abandoned

Countering Depression with Positive Thoughts and Actions

This book can also help you stay positive. Almost every chapter, beginning with the first, offers concrete ways to counter depression by living a full life that is active, engaged, and intentional and sings with independence. It isn't the same as your pre-dementia life, but I believe with a focus on the positive side of living with dementia, it can be a very good life. Having a "bucket list," finding things that make you happy, letting go, laughing at yourself, creating a supportive environment, communicating more effectively—these all speak to countering depression by living completely and not holding back. In an automatic, natural manner, your mind will find it difficult to hold onto the feelings of depression as you take the steps to live fully and positively at the same time. The good news here is that research suggests people with dementia are less likely to develop more symptoms of depression but rather, to become less depressed over time.

A wealth of online materials for you and your caregivers describe suggested treatments for depression in people living with dementia. Please visit healthline.com or familydoctor.org for more information. I sincerely hope you are not experiencing symptoms of depression but if you are, my heart goes out to you. Dementia is not the only potential cause of depression in the elderly. Both the normal changes in lifestyle associated with aging and living in long-term residential care are potent contributors. Are these factors relevant for you? If so and you are feeling depressed, they may be part of the problem.

Don't Forgot Your Care Partners

Finally, you are not alone in your battle with depression. Your caregivers may also be struggling with it as well. It is estimated that 30 to 50 percent of Alzheimer's caregivers, especially the primary caregivers, will experience depression during your lifetime, in part as the result of the changes in their lives that result from caring for you. This is one of the reasons why having a caregiver team is so important to your health and their health. Other factors that will make a big difference and reduce their burden are your positive attitude, your choice to live a full life, and your independence.

KEY POINTS

- Finding moments of happiness, every day, in your life with dementia is one of the keys to living a full life. People who are happy are also healthier, live longer, and have more social support.

- Happiness, to a large degree, depends on choices you make. Because much of the reality you experience is created in your mind, you will decide whether to find and interpret events in a way that adds joy to your life—or not.

- Life with dementia can be filled with moments of uncertainty and frustration when things don't work as well as expected. Add health and happiness by learning "not to sweat the small stuff." Release the negativity in these moments, accept them, and move on.

- A focus on finding joyful moments and happiness can add thousands of hours of positive, quality time to your life.

- Depression can be part of your experience with dementia, especially in the early stages. If you are feeling depressed, seek help from your caregivers, health professionals, and the excellent materials published by the Alzheimer's community.

- Your happiness is important to your care partners. By choosing to find moments of joy every day in your life, you are supporting these partners by making their lives happier and healthier.

Ideas for your life? How might you act on them? What is the first step?

3

Embrace the Story of Your Life

For that dash represents all the time that they spent alive on earth. And now only those who loved them know what that little line is worth. For it matters not, how much we own, the cars . . . the house . . . the cash. What matters is how we live and love and how we spend our dash.

—Linda Ellis, "The Dash"

Every life tells a story, a story filled with many chapters that include your childhood, education, career, friendships, and loves, your adventures, and, no less important, your biggest challenges, hardships, and failures. Each of us remembers many parts of our story—but it's an incomplete memory, with research suggesting that the high points and low points are the most likely to be recalled, while the time or *meantime* in between is largely a blur. In fact, when we look back at the significant events in our life, our recollections are often reduced to two components: the core part of the event and the ending or outcome. Most other details vanished long ago from our conscious minds. Because endings are so important to us, it makes the ending of our story very significant, long before it occurs.

The content of your life story speaks not just to the events described above and their outcomes but also to how *you* experienced them. Were you strong and courageous, passive and weak, leader or follower, vulnerable or stoic, forward-thinking or history-bound—or a dozen other things? Did you accomplish much of what you set out to do in life or watch in frustration as others who were more successful passed you by? Who are the other characters in this story?—a spouse? children, grandchildren? friends? It is likely that much of your story is part of a collective memory, a chronological history shared by these other characters. As you leave this history behind, they will often struggle to maintain it.

What does a diagnosis of Alzheimer's do to your story? Does discovering the Dementia Card work like the Go to Jail Card in Monopoly, bringing your journey in pursuit of happiness to a close? Or does it just pause it for a moment until you begin the process of living fully again, but with dementia? Finally, what about the ending—an important part of any story? How will your ending with Alzheimer's differ from the ending you were planning?

Helping with Direction

Your life story is a ribbon, stretching across time, that captures the essence of your personal history in encapsulated form and gives it a structure. Think of the story as the elevator speech of this history, describing in just a few words the major events in your life. It also offers, as I think you will discover, a powerful set of landmarks to navigate by in your Alzheimer's journey. If you are struggling now with a new diagnosis, wondering what to do next, your story can help ground you and point your spinning compass in the right direction.

Every story has a theme based on your life history, personality, and choices you have made. It is the theme that ties together the many events in your life and gives them structure and meaning in time. Without the theme, it may be difficult for others to follow the events in your life and connect them in a way that makes sense. Perhaps the story is about your success in overcoming the odds to go from rags to riches, or from being unknown to becoming a star. Perhaps it is about love—love of another person, love of adventure, passion in your art or work. Perhaps it is about a struggle for a cause, for your rights as a person of color, against gender inequality or sexual bias, or for the environment. There are many possible themes and your choice determines the type of story that you are living.

The end of your story, set in the future, is just a concept at this point, not reality. It is an important concept, however, because thinking about this ending influences your expectations in a way that affects the present. In today's fear-based Alzheimer's culture, there are few good examples of positive endings, because *the stories about these endings come from caregivers and physicians, not the person.* Yet you will want to find a way to be comfortable with how you view the end of your story, to help it support your living life fully with Alzheimer's now. What is an ending that makes sense, given your story's theme? We will come back to this important topic in a later chapter.

A Second Chance

Perhaps the biggest change in your story is that it has a new chapter titled something like "Living with Dementia." It's a difficult chapter to write because, even after you choose to live fully, some of what you will experience will be negative. In part this is because the context (how the world views dementia) is often negative, and also because you will face many challenges as your own reality diverges from the reality of your caregivers. Given this fact, it would be difficult not to feel some anxiety over the changes in your mind you can see happening now and what you can anticipate for the future.

Imagine for a moment that you are given a second chance. Your physician calls in the morning and informs you that the Alzheimer's diagnosis was a mistake. Instead of Alzheimer's, you have a mild form of dementia with similar symptoms but without the long-term effects. You will experience some muddled thinking, occasional speech problems, and memory loss, but it will be more benign, a process similar to what happens to many people as they age. If you take the pill he will prescribe, many of these symptoms will vanish.

How would you react to this news? Would you breathe a sigh of relief and prepare (with your family) to go on living, knowing that the mild dementia will be an inconvenience but one you can handle? Would you look forward to the future, knowing there were many good moments to come, that life as you know it is not over? Would your attitude shift from grief and anxiety to acceptance? Would you rely on the mental toughness we all learn to develop as we age and our bodies and minds undergo natural changes? Would your story go back to being the one you have been writing for many years—with a few new bumps?

If the answer is "yes," then perhaps you can see the negative power that an Alzheimer's diagnosis carries. It is negative because *it confounds hope for curing the disease with hope for living fully and joyfully.* When it takes away the latter, it can quickly dampen your optimism about the future. Just as you could see in the above example how reversing the Alzheimer's diagnosis would quickly alter your story, you can also understand how changing your attitude can change your story now. The only way you will give grief and misery control over the next 10 years of your life is by clinging to the false reality that the Alzheimer's myth represents, the belief that joy in your life is over. Reality is not an immutable hunk of rock; it is based on the interaction of your mind and the world. You have a voice in creating the reality that you want.

Your Story Living with Dementia/Alzheimer's

Part of the dementia community intentionally approaches the disease in a negative way because fear, grief, and the inconvenience of life with Alzheimer's are the primary drivers of fundraising. A workshop offered nationally on Alzheimer's and dementia in the spring of 2015 by Frank Sesno of Georgetown University used the following program description: "When the diagnosis is Alzheimer's disease or dementia, grief doesn't wait for death. Grieving can begin in the doctor's office when patients and families receive the news (and span the next decade)."

If your current story has picked up this negative attitude, my heart goes out to you. You can take a more positive path, one that will serve you much better.

The reality is that dementia doesn't suddenly bring your previous life story to a dramatic, negative end. It does change things. It does add another chapter that will affect your life in significant ways, and many of these are negative. Like any disorder, mental or physical, it is likely to add inconvenience and some pain to your life. It's not the same story of aging in the traditional ways you expected, even though the physical ending may be similar.

Richard Taylor adds his perspective here: *"I am starting to fear the coming end of me. Not the death of me but the end of me as I know myself and others know me."*

If the old story is no longer valid, and you elect not to adopt the negative perspective common to much of the Alzheimer's community for your next chapter, what are your options? You could try the Pollyanna approach and claim the next chapter will be a piece of cake, but neither you nor anyone else believes this.

The answer is pretty straightforward: You build this next chapter of your story around living fully but realistically with dementia, planning your future and taking the steps you need to make your life as happy as possible.

It is true that your physician can't offer you a cure, but not being cured of an illness and living a full life are very different subjects. Part of the mystique of Alzheimer's is that many aspects are negative for you and for your family. But consider for a moment, what is positive about a broken leg, cancer, or any other medical problem? Not very much. The question for you is pretty clear: Are you willing to sacrifice the quality of the remainder of your life to maintain the integrity of the old story? I certainly hope not.

Now you can see the relevance of the choices you made earlier. If you choose to find ways to be happy, whenever possible, despite the inconvenience Alzheimer's or other forms of dementia will bring, you will have a story that for many years will be dominated by positive experiences.

One purpose of this book is to help send you on the Alzheimer's journey with a different perspective and accompanied by a new story. You need a story that moves from grieving to acceptance of your new life; a story focused on the positive side of what you will experience, not the negative; and finally, a story in which you find a way to live a complete and joyful life.

If this sounds like a total fantasy, look around you. Read the stories and blogs of those who have lived many years with dementia in a positive way. Look at the caregiver stories that speak not to the pain and inconvenience of dementia care but to the personhood and well-being that are maintained throughout the process. Finally, imagine the power of giving your story a slight twist (as I just did) by switching the Alzheimer's diagnosis to one of mild dementia. Use this power to give your life with Alzheimer's a positive outlook. Receiving an Alzheimer's diagnosis is not a good thing, but when that becomes your new story, good and bad from the perspective of the "old story" do not matter. It is time to move on.

A significant part of every story is the ending. How will Alzheimer's change the ending of your story? Perhaps not as much as you might think.

A New Ending

As we look to the future, most of us have at least a rough idea of how we would like our story to end. Reality might discourage us if we fully understood the frailty of the human body and mind; nevertheless, in our minds, a good story has a good ending. While we know death is certain, we expect to maintain a good life, with the inconvenience of gradual decline, for many years to come. In our world and culture at this time, this is what we have come to anticipate. If family and friends are present to provide support and help when needed, so much the better. That's an acceptable way for the story to end. Other less-ideal endings are possible—a battle with cancer, a sudden heart attack, an accident—but in every case, the story has a natural ending.

Here are some recent examples of endings from several obituaries:

The Master Electrician dimmed the light on the life of George HA, a retired electrical engineer, on Thursday, Oct. 1, 2015.

Wiley GJB, 88, a loving husband, father, grandfather and friend, passed away Sunday, Oct. 4, 2015.

Donald RS, a theater producer in New York and London who became a civic leader in Boston, died on Sept. 30 at his home there. He was 103.

Margaret A, age 82, died peacefully surrounded by family on Saturday, Oct. 10, 2015, at the home of her daughter, DA.

Do these sound real to you? I don't think so! These kinds of obituaries are basically myths designed to put a good face on death and what preceded it. A common theme in these accounts is the good fight or brave battle against disease. Such endings belong more to the medical establishment and its need to extend life at any cost than to the individuals involved. Yes, you are a fighter. That's great, but it can also lead to a great deal of unnecessary misery when there is little point to doing battle.

Perhaps the most common ending theme, illustrated above, is some version of "died comfortably in her sleep surrounded by family and friends." This happens occasionally I'm sure, although I know of few comfortable deaths. My parents and grandparents did not experience this kind of ending. Dr. Angelo Volandes, an end-of-life expert at Harvard Medical School, points out the real statistics: More than half of deaths take place in hospitals, not the home—and last-minute interventions to extend life make up one-third of Medicare costs! The fiction of a good death does make a good story, however, and one that sets up expectations for others about how they would like their story to end.

Preserving the Family History

A person nearing the end of life has, in most cultures, a significant role to play as the keeper of precious family knowledge, wisdom, history, and wishes that might be passed on to the next generation or to close family and friends. To fulfill this role, you will not want to wait much longer, whether you choose to act directly now or to create letters or other materials that will be opened at your death. At the moment, you have some control over what is to be shared, but this may not last much longer.

As you tell your story and create your personal history to be used as part of your digital "companion mind" (described in a later chapter), be aware that this history contains information that you may want to share with future generations. Keep this in mind as you work with your caregivers to decide what to collect. Your primary goal is to gather things to support your journey, but in the future, others may view this digital mind as a representation of you and your life. You may also want to visit one of the online sites, such as ancestry.com, that are set up to keep many parts of this history intact and accessible to others.

I've always loved the concept of time capsules that share something from today's world with future generations. Now is the time to create your own time capsule to share what is on your mind with your family. It will serve to document your life and wishes in a manner that can help you to end your story on your own terms.

Despite what you may think, your eventual death with Alzheimer's is likely to be similar to the deaths of everyone else, not necessarily easy or convenient but pretty normal and tied to one of the many conditions that afflict us as we age. Dying with Alzheimer's is mostly about dying as you age—with complications. The disease and its impact on systems regulated by your brain can complicate things, but in this fluid, uncertain time, separating the impact of Alzheimer's from that of aging and other possible issues is not easy. If the ending will be normal, then what matters most is the second part of your story about how you spend your time between now and that eventual death. That is the core.

KEY POINTS

- Your life tells a story filled with many adventures, loves, successes, failures, and much more. Each of us tends to remember the highs and lows while the "normal time" in between is often more blurred. We remember not just the events but also how we felt about them or experienced them.

- Alzheimer's changes your story because it changes your experience now, in the present, and also the ending. Or does it? Actually, the main themes of your story were established many years ago. These themes, based on your personal history, will play a crucial role in guiding you as you live with dementia; they will also influence how others relate to you.

- Your new story, living with dementia, is not the fearful, negative one promoted today in the Alzheimer's community. Instead, given your choice in Chapter 1, it is just a new chapter in the old story with new challenges, opportunities, and adventures.

- You are not holding your breath while we wait for a cure but rather seeking the path that allows you to live fully but realistically with dementia, using all of the tools and technology that are available today. This book is full of help for you.

- The lives of other individuals, such as Rick Phelps or Brian LeBlanc, who are living a full life despite an Alzheimer's diagnosis can help you understand the full range of possibilities still open for you and your life.

- Remember that your personal history is an irreplaceable treasure in the context of your family's history. You may want to take the steps now, in the early stages of dementia, to preserve as much of this history (and your story) as possible for others.

Ideas for your life? How might you act on them? What is the first step?

4

Living with Hope: Rethinking Aging

The process of fighting off symptoms is exhausting, and yet exhilarating when I succeed.

—Greg O'Brien, *On Pluto: Inside the Mind of Alzheimer's*

In the previous chapter, I asked you to go back in time to a point before the Alzheimer's diagnosis and imagine what your story might be like. How would your attitude about life change if you didn't realize you had the disease? A remarkable body of research on nuns and Alzheimer's disease reported by D.A Bennett in "Selected Findings from The Religious Order Study and the Rush Memory and Aging Project" in the *Journal of Alzheimer's Disease* has been looking at a population of Catholic nuns since 1986. The ongoing study gives us some insight into how your attitude might change things. The nuns were part of a large study on aging and cognitive skills. For many years, they were regularly given comprehensive tests to evaluate their ability to perform basic memory functions and other mental skills. These tests continued until their deaths and then their brains were examined to see if physical damage to the brain could be related to cognitive function.

Some of the results were unexpected and quite amazing. Many nuns in the study had brains showing significant damage due to Alzheimer's disease, while their performance on a battery of cognitive tests was normal! Let me repeat that finding. Many nuns with full-blown, late-stage Alzheimer's were not aware of it, because they were living a normal life. The annual tests they took did not show the decline in mental skills we might associate with the disease. The statistics showed that only 25 percent of the variability in cognitive functioning could be attributed to dementia or other disorders. How can this be?

To answer this question, I want you to consider several concepts that contributed to this remarkable finding.

Living Life Fully: Resilient Aging

We can view the decline in cognitive functioning with Alzheimer's as a process that we cannot change or slow significantly without the magic pill that will provide a cure. Or, we can see the changes in function as something we can definitely influence. We can embrace the flexibility in our lifestyles and our attitudes, combine this with an understanding of the plasticity in the architecture of our brains, and try on the notion that reality is, in large part, a fiction created by our minds. The nuns in this study lived a full physical, mental, and spiritual life with exercise; mental games such as bridge, Scrabble, and crossword puzzles; and prayer as part of their regular routine. They lived a life that by today's standards for aging was probably less stressful than most, because of the presence of long-term "family" connections, a supportive environment, and familiar routines.

Lifestyle Factors that Might Support Resilient Aging

- Low-stress environment with physical and economic security
- A healthy diet
- Regular physical exercise
- Mental stimulation with puzzles and games
- Established routines and habits
- Prayer and meditation
- Regular singing
- Strong, supportive social community
- Living for others—people outside of themselves to focus on and provide love and support
- Nurturing atmosphere that is likely to reduce the emphasis on ego and testing

Some combination of these and other factors leads to "resilient aging," or aging in a manner that promotes the flexibility of the brain to respond to neurodegenerative diseases such as Alzheimer's. Many recent studies show the power of diet, exercise, and mental stimulation in this context, so we might assume these factors are part of a healthy lifestyle. I will come back to this important topic in a later chapter.

Cognitive Reserve

How can a person with advanced Alzheimer's have normal cognitive functioning? How is this possible, when a large percentage of the neurons and the circuits they create to define our intelligence are destroyed? The answer is cognitive reserve. Put simply, redundancies in the brain allow other parts of the brain to take over to replace the damaged areas. Some people have enough cognitive reserve to tolerate the damage caused by dementia without developing clear clinical symptoms.

Think about this fact for a moment. What it means is that some people with Alzheimer's are living normal lives today because they have sufficient cognitive reserve to overcome the disabilities the disease often causes. How do you increase your cognitive reserve? Research suggests that cognitive reserve is enhanced by a lifetime experience that includes higher levels of education, more social interaction, and more cognitive stimulation.

How much cognitive reserve do you have? Not quite enough to eliminate all symptoms of Alzheimer's, otherwise you wouldn't be reading this book. But you can see that creating more cognitive reserve with a change in attitude or lifestyle may significantly influence the quality of your life in the future. There is hope for improving your life with dementia that depends on things you can control.

Dementia puts the most pressure on left-brain functions, such as speaking, reasoning, and judgment-based activities. Your right-brain functions—the creative, holistic, image-oriented part of your mind—will remain more intact and form the core of your cognitive reserve "bank." The activities described in several later chapters offer a path for keeping your mental account balance healthy.

Dementia and Aging: A New Perspective

As you can see from the nuns research, it is possible to have advanced Alzheimer's without having the typical symptoms. On the other hand, many people have the symptoms of Alzheimer's without having the disease. A simple diagram from this research illustrates these options in the context of dementia and aging.

Chart 4A

	No Pathology	Pathology
Normal Cognition	**HEALTHY AGING** No Symptoms	**RESILIENT AGING** No Symptoms
Abnormal Cognition	**COGNITIVELY FRAIL AGING** Dementia Symptoms	**DEMENTIA** Dementia Symptoms

The shift in thinking is based on what has been observed in the population of aging adults. Symptoms of dementia are not always based on having a brain with dementia but may be part of a normal aging process. (My dad had mild dementia for several years but did not have Alzheimer's or other types of brain damage associated with dementia.) All three of the light-gray boxes above offer opportunities for a somewhat normal life. The Resilient Aging box reminds us that developing a more plastic brain supports living with dementia without showing major symptoms. The Cognitively Frail box reminds us that many people with symptoms of dementia do not have the disease; instead, the symptoms are a function of aging.

It may be possible to reduce the symptoms of dementia with changes in lifestyle, medications, and so on with and without having the disease. As you can see, this is a very flexible, fluid space where your experience of dementia can change over time. Currently, your Alzheimer's diagnosis means that you do have the symptoms of dementia. It doesn't guarantee that those symptoms aren't due to aging, or that due to your cognitive reserve, they can't be reduced over time.

I think a different diagram is needed to illustrate what is happening here. Let's focus just on the symptoms of dementia, since that's what is concerning you today.

Chart 4B

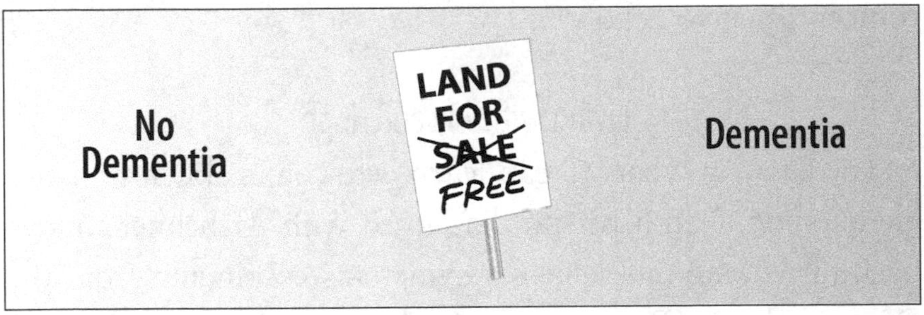

No Boundaries

What the research on dementia teaches us is that the boundaries in Figure 4A are misleading. The territory between dementia and no dementia is vast and filled with ambiguity. Much of this territory is unclaimed. What are the boundaries of age-related dementia with no pathology involved? No one knows definitively. What is the range of behavior for someone with Alzheimer's that could extend into this middle zone? That is also not clear.

Research on mental activities such as crossword puzzles or word games illustrates the importance of this middle zone. The results of these studies make it very clear that while such activities will not prevent the eventual decline in cognitive functioning that comes with Alzheimer's, they do *delay* this decline—capturing many precious, positive moments in time.

What is apparent here is that the concept of dementia, and the boundaries between no dementia and advanced dementia, are fluid and filled with shades of gray. That is good news. This is territory you might grab with the latest medications, changes in lifestyle, and a dozen other things described in this book. This is the territory that is influenced by the choices you make, the acceptance and love of your family members, and the environments that you choose.

Living with Joy and Hope

The heart of what we can learn here comes down to a single question. Can a person diagnosed with Alzheimer's move backward along the dementia symptoms continuum from the Dementia box in Figure 4A to the Resilient Mind box? Both of these boxes represent individuals with physical damage to their brains due to dementia, but very different lives. We don't know the answer, but you can imagine the potential if the answer was "yes" and you had the power to affect some of the symptoms you are experiencing.

Remember the exercise where I asked you to imagine going back in time to a point before the Alzheimer's diagnosis? If you could go back to this place and use everything you could learn about developing a lifestyle to support Resilient Aging to move yourself in this direction, would you do it? In other words, despite having the symptoms of dementia and a diagnosis of Alzheimer's, would you consider *leaving* the Dementia category for Resilient Aging? In a heartbeat you would! Then I would say that based on all we know you need to try. As Figure 4B illustrates, the four boxes in Figure 4A are not really fixed. There are large areas of unclaimed territory between them. Go for it!

Meditation and Dementia

Meditation has been shown to have a profound effect on the physical structure of the human brain and the neuronal activity patterns it generates. The nuns in the study described above all engage regularly in meditative prayer as part of their daily experience. Could this be a clue that might help you move from the Dementia box to Resilient Aging? At this time, there is no experimental evidence for this because the research has not been done. The hints coming from studies in non-dementia populations are very suggestive. More about this topic later.

What about current medicines or treatment techniques? Do they offer hope? The next chapter addresses this important subject.

KEY POINTS

- Amazing research on a population of nuns demonstrates that some people with Alzheimer's are not aware of the disease because they are living a normal life. Three factors can help us understand this remarkable discovery.

  Resilient aging: This is aging in a manner that promotes the flexibility of the brain to respond to neurodegenerative diseases. Diet, exercise, and a number of other factors appear to make this more likely to occur in individuals.

  Cognitive reserve: Some brains have redundancies that, when parts of the brain are damaged by dementia, permit other parts to take over the functions of the damaged areas.

  Dementia symptoms and aging: Some symptoms of dementia can appear as a normal part of the healthy aging process without the presence of the disease.

- The territory between dementia and non-dementia is vast and filled with ambiguity. Much of this territory is unclaimed. What are the boundaries of age-related dementia with no pathology involved? No one knows definitively. To what extent can you, living with dementia, claim new territory in the land of non-dementia based on resilient aging? No one knows.

- Living a full life means pushing the boundaries to benefit from cognitive reserve and resilient aging whenever possible. Meditation may be one behavior that can help. The lifestyles of the nuns used in this research also suggest many other possibilities.

Ideas for your life? How might you act on them? What is the first step?

5

Taking Your Medicine

You have to row harder with dementia or you drift.

Sure, there are many who encourage from the shoreline: family, friends, doctors, and colleagues, many of them not fully understanding why they are waving. In Alzheimer's, one is in the boat alone. So, you row a little harder!

—Greg O'Brien, *On Pluto: Inside the Mind of Alzheimer's*

While there is no cure for dementia today, there may be a cure available in the next few years that could significantly reduce the impact of the disease and improve the quality of your life. I sincerely hope this happens—and quickly. Living fully with Alzheimer's means embracing the possibility that today's sophisticated medical science will offer you this hope.

Billions of dollars are invested each year in finding a cure, as well as in developing preventive measures, methods for early detection, and ways to delay the progression of the disease once it has been diagnosed. Some recent research offers promise here, but still no pill and no treatment hits the jackpot.

If you are being treated by a physician, it is likely that you are taking pills of some sort to help slow the symptoms of the disease. Medicine, even if it doesn't yet work well, does three important things.

1. It offers you the hope of extending the time that your mind functions in a fairly normal manner, so you can add quality moments with the people and things that you love.

2. It offers your physicians a partial answer to their current helplessness when it comes to treating Alzheimer's. Pills and surgery are the backbone of conventional health care. Now your doctor can say, "Take two of these a day."

3. It offers your family and other caregivers a respite from their perceived helplessness. Now at least there is something concrete they can give you that has potential. Even if it is little more than a Band-Aid, it represents progress.

Small Improvements Are a Big Deal

You may be wondering why I am describing a treatment option that at the moment doesn't work well for most people. In the context of this book—living life to its fullest with Alzheimer's—there are two answers to this question. The first is that small improvements are big gains when it comes to treating Alzheimer's disease. The promises for available medicines today (like the many TV ads you see for treatments for other diseases) tend to be exaggerated, but they still offer some help. In our terms, they offer more positive, quality moments—and those long moments are always precious.

The second answer is more important. Most of this book encourages you to accept your diagnosis, live with it, and find positive ways to move on with your life. This chapter is here to remind you not to give up hope for help from the medical community at any point along the journey.

New understanding—of how Alzheimer's damages the brain, which areas are affected, how to prevent this, and how to reverse it—is coming rapidly now. Results from several major research studies offer the possibility of a major breakthrough. Interested in helping by being a participant in research? The National Institute on Aging is currently looking for 70,000 volunteers to participate in over 150 studies! There is no guarantee of a solution, but at the same time, there is reason to hope—and I want that hope to be part of the toolkit you take with you on your Alzheimer's journey.

Dementia, like most disorders, has its share of magic cures, natural-ingredients-that-can-solve-any-problem, and a variety of alternative approaches with mixed results. Some of these may have considerable value. Some are probably quackery. Before becoming invested in any of these approaches, I suggest you consult with your care partners and physicians to get a second opinion. Unfortunately, today's seniors are the target of many health-related scams and, despite your dementia, you are no exception.

The Magic of Sleep: Can It Offer Hope Now?

Living with a diagnosis of Alzheimer's means that no pill that you can take right now is likely to prevent it. That would be magic. However, recent brain research does offer some exciting possibilities about one potential cause of dementia and something you can do now that may slow its progression. In the future, I think this discovery will also be one key to preventing Alzheimer's.

What is this remarkable new finding? Let me give you a brief analogy before I describe it. Think of your dishwasher. All day long, it collects dirty dishes and if, like me, you don't do a good job of rinsing, they are covered with food particles. After dinner, you add soap, push the "on" button and presto, in an hour, the dishes are clean with all the waste flushed away.

The glymphatic system in your brain operates in a similar manner. At night, while you are sleeping, it sends a fluid through your brain that picks up the wastes from brain tissue—in particular discarded proteins such as the beta-amyloid peptides that are associated with Alzheimer's—and flushes them from your head. For this flushing process to work efficiently, however, one thing is crucial. You must be asleep! People with sleep disorders do not get the full benefit of this cleansing activity, leaving many of the discarded proteins in the brain.

Does this one process explain the cause of Alzheimer's disease? I think that is unlikely, although the process could be a core part of the mechanism. What it does suggest is a simple and powerful way of delaying the symptoms of dementia that, in the future, may be a key part of every treatment program: the magic of sleep.

It is a well-known fact that people who sleep poorly are more likely to get Alzheimer's disease or other forms of dementia. The glymphatic research suggests there may be a causal relationship here, since less sleep means less effective flushing of unwanted waste proteins.

Since you are living with Alzheimer's, *preventing* dementia doesn't concern us at the moment. But what if a key future treatment for people with dementia involved more effective cleansing of the brain to slow or stop the progression of the disease? There is no guarantee here and certainly no drugs or treatment process available to do this. However, there is one simple thing you can do right now that can help. Sleep. Sleep more. Sleep well. More and better sleep, according to neuroscientists Steven Goldman and Maiken Nedergaard, is associated with more complete flushing of unwanted products from the brain—products that are linked to dementia.

Pills that can help you sleep well may help slow the onset of dementia and may, in the future, be a key part of a treatment program.

Richard Taylor was always pessimistic about the potential of pills to help but was wise enough to take them. Here is his humorous perspective on the chances for a major discovery that could be of benefit:

I have stopped reading about the "breakthroughs" in research on Alzheimer's disease that appear so frequently in the popular press. If they find what causes it, how to stop it, how to reverse the damage it causes to healthy brains, then I'll buy the special issue of Time *magazine and read it.*

Today you will find the news on Twitter and Facebook first, I am sure! Richard was a wise and courageous person who lived his life to the fullest and, while he was skeptical about the chances for a cure in his lifetime, he never gave up hope.

KEY POINTS

- While there is currently no cure for Alzheimer's or procedure that significantly delays its onset, billions are being spent each year looking for such solutions.

- Current medications can offer limited help and may add many positive, quality moments to your life. Small improvements are big gains when it comes to treating dementia.

- The potential of new discoveries, in your lifetime, offers hope that you can receive help at a future time. In the meantime, your best strategy is to focus on finding ways to live well with your disability.

- Recent research suggests that the glymphatic system, which flushes harmful wastes associated with Alzheimer's from your brain tissues while you sleep, could a key factor in preventing or slowing the onset of dementia. This research highlights the importance of getting a good night's sleep.

- People with dementia often do not sleep well. This may or may not apply to you. However, doing what it takes to sleep longer and more deeply might be beneficial.

- Waste no opportunity in your battle with dementia. Take your medicine!

Ideas for your life? How might you act on them? What is the first step?

6

Embarking on a Hero's Journey

I wanted others to know that they are not alone with an Alzheimer's chang-
ing mind. There are others with them on the Alzheimer's road less traveled who
are uneasy about the present and the future, and unable to figure things out as
they have in the past.

—Richard Taylor, *Alzheimer's Inside Out*

The Alzheimer's process is a journey. I call it a "Hero's Journey" because you will leave Earth-reality, a familiar land of
words, concepts, and people with whom you share much in
common, and travel to a new planet named Altzair. I introduced
the idea of a special planet in my previous book as a way of
explaining that Alzheimer's does not simply give you a modified
view of Earth-reality but, instead, takes you to a completely
different planet. Greg O'Brien uses the planet Pluto to describe
his experiences with dementia in his book, *On Pluto: Inside the*
Mind of Alzheimer's.

The stages in your journey are well-known but not well understood, because the clinical descriptions tied to early-, mid-, and
late-stage Alzheimer's cannot do justice to the complexity and
richness of what is happening in your conscious mind. The first
part of your journey is likely to take you from the left-brained

world of logic and language to one dominated by heart and emotions. As you make this transition, you may find it frustrating at times. Your caregivers and friends will not always follow quickly enough to understand your new perspective. Richard Taylor describes his experience here:

The locus of my attention is definitely shifting from my head to my heart. I feel and think about feelings more than I think about thinking. I feel sad, and mad, and happy, and grateful. I feel loved, ignored, needed, and like a dying albatross that is chained around each of the people who care about me.

Courage Is Required

No one makes the Alzheimer's journey by choice. It's a mission driven by heredity, lifestyle, fate, and certainly age. To make this journey successfully and continue to live a full life while you are traveling, courage is required. You must be ready to confront and challenge the reality of your life with the disease, armed with all the tools that are available.

The next stage of your journey will probably leave behind the familiar boundaries of time as your mind and memory begin to disconnect from past and future, suspending you in the present tense. As you may see, the idea of "living in the present" or "being here now" takes on a whole new meaning in this context. Being stranded in the present means that you "let go" of the normal tendency to connect the moment with future and past, but it also opens the door for you to experience many meaningful, joyful long moments.

One of the biggest challenges you are likely to face is getting information from others on the nature of this journey. This book, with its stories and content based on the accounts of others with Alzheimer's, may help, but the truth is that no one with advanced dementia has ever returned to give us a full report. Also, while no two journeys will be the same, there is a wealth of information, beyond what I describe in this book, offered by organizations such as the Dementia Alliance International (dementiaallianceinternational.org) and Dementia Action Alliance (daanow.org) that may help.

The Planet Altzair

Eventually, most travelers with Alzheimer's will reach the planet Altzair, the land of dreams, where what is happening in your mind is much like a dream—a private reality that belongs only to you. Now, just as at your birth, what remains is your core consciousness of light and spirit, and your essence as a human being. Visitors who come hoping to find the old landscape of your history with them will be disappointed. Those who embrace your heart and spirit and accept that you now live on a different world they cannot understand will give you much comfort.

You already know that growing old can be pretty challenging. Physical and mental skills that you took for granted most of your life may no longer be accessible. Visits to the dentist or the doctor for care often require tests and treatments that are no fun. Your independence as a person can suffer as you become more dependent on others for your care. This is just a normal part of aging and, managed well, has little to do with the quality of your life.

Given your dementia diagnosis, the journey you are beginning is not a negative experience or a thing to be feared. It is just your reality, in the same way that radiation treatments, wheelchairs, incontinence, and incurable cancer are realities for others. You already understand that it's an arduous journey that may test you in many ways, because no one gives up Earth-reality without a battle.

Companions on Your Journey

Your allies and companions on this journey will be your care partners. The journey is likely to also test them. The emotions that you will all experience—the love, the pain, the grief, the frustration and uncertainty—can challenge you with their immediacy and intensity. They can also reward you in many ways as you move past the everyday chatter in your mind to quiet understanding and acceptance.

This is a journey that you will largely make alone. Your friends and caregivers can see you, hear you, and interact with you, but they can share only to a very limited degree what is happening in your consciousness. Your caregiver companions who learn to "come to you" during the journey will be precious allies and the source of many long moments of joy and comfort. Even better, they are not just present for your comfort. As you will see in later chapters, they can become expert guides who will support you with clear communication, non-judgment, and constructive guidance. Their knowledge can damp the flames of confusion and frustration you will experience at times as the boundaries of Earth-reality no longer fit your own world.

Later I will introduce the idea of adding a new kind of companion to your caregiver team: a digital partner who is familiar with your life history and can work with you 24/7 to provide entertainment, information, and support. There is no reason that today's marvelous technology for teenagers cannot be adapted in creative, useful ways to fit the elderly and to support your challenges in living with dementia.

Remember that throughout the journey, you will still always be you. You were born a whole person and you will live your life as a complete, whole person—even when the rest of the world no longer recognizes you in the cloak of Alzheimer's. Your song will always be loud and clear. The essence of you, your life, and your spirit will always be present in the hearts and minds of those people whom you hold close.

I know you may be afraid of this journey. There is much that we don't understand about dementia. I also know that while the journey is not voluntary (you would have selected another path, given the option), now that you have made the choice to live a full and joyful life, that is the life you will find. I believe the hero in you is up to the challenge.

It may seem like a small step to view Alzheimer's and your journey in a positive manner, but this is not the case. When you make this choice and the choice to seek happiness wherever you can find it, you open a whole universe of options that will feed you thousands of moments of joy, peace, and normality.

This small book offers a number of tools and ideas to help you and your caregivers add joyful, quality moments. Our focus is on a single goal for you: *continuing the parade.*

My heart goes out to you as you begin your journey. I will listen for your song.

KEY POINTS

- The Alzheimer's process is a journey from a familiar land of words and an Earth-reality that is shared with family and friends to a new planet called Altzair. It is similar in many ways to the "hero's journey" described by pioneering psychologist Carl Jung.

- Your core being of heart and spirit along with your identity as a person will make this journey—but it will challenge your independence and your courage.

- It is a journey you must make largely alone. Your care partners and others can be companions but, once the journey begins, you cannot return to their world any more than they can enter yours.

- These partners will need to learn to "come to you" during the journey with communication and support instead of testing or attempting to pull you back into Earth-reality.

- By choosing to live fully and continue your parade, you will find many people and opportunities along the way that can offer help and add joy to your life.

Ideas for your life? How might you act on them? What is the first step?

PREPARING FOR THE JOURNEY

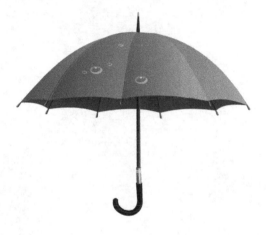

7

Lessons from Aging: What Makes Life Worth Living?

What I need to feel is that I am still taking care of something. Something that returns love, that gives itself away without expecting anything back, that wants to please me ... all the time!

—Richard Taylor, from his blog article,
"Why Plants Make the Best Pets"

The Alzheimer's journey is a story about dementia, but at its heart it is also about aging. As you read this book, unless you have early-onset dementia, you are likely to be in your 70s, 80s, or 90s. How you live your life now will be defined by many of the same factors important to anyone who is elderly. Ultimately, with or without dementia, much of the quality of your life and your well-being will depend on these factors.

What are the things that make life worth living? Good question. If we look at the last 10 years of life for people in almost every setting (living at home or in an institution; with almost any kind of health problem, ranging from none to cancer or Parkinson's disease; and with almost any lifestyle, from being alone to being surrounded by family), the core things that matter most to ensure a quality life are roughly the same.

What about people with Alzheimer's? Surely the same rules don't apply. Actually, they do. Dementia may change the way you define "independence" (important to everyone) but the concept remains the same. In fact, with memory loss, maintaining a degree of independence is essential to your well-being.

What are the keys to living a quality life as we age? In almost every study, the following four factors stand out:

1. Personal: achieving independence and self-competence
2. Social: forming connections with others
3. Physical: having a supportive physical environment
4. Spiritual: finding meaning by living for others

Let's look more carefully at each of these factors in the context of what you will be experiencing with Alzheimer's.

Personal independence. Your ability to have some control over the important dimensions of your life is especially important in the early and middle stages. You will be functioning normally to a large degree and will want your independence as an adult to be respected by your family, friends, and caregivers. (Several chapters in this book, especially the chapters on personhood and communication, offer help here.) Early on, every bit of independence you can maintain is precious for your health. In later stages, your sense of independence will depend on your caregivers' willingness to understand and respect your personhood, and the steps they take to support you as an adult.

Connections with friends and family. Many different social models work fine to meet this need. You can have a network of connections with friends, family, and caregivers, or you can be connected with a single caregiver, spouse, or friend. The key is to have some form of social support and regular social contact.

Organizations such as the Alzheimer's Society (dementiafriends. org) and Dementia Action Alliance (daanow.org) offer great resources for those who might not otherwise have a healthy social life.

A friendly environment. A key part of living a good life as an older person with dementia is having the good fortune to live in a safe and friendly environment. What does this mean? Friendly environments are ones where: the furniture is accessible and designed for easy use; the tools needed to support everyday functions, such as dressing, bathing, dining, and sleeping, are clearly marked and accessible; pathways and locations are easily identified and clearly marked, when required; and the treatment of light, color, and space adds a livable, esthetic quality.

Environments that support assisted living go hand-in-hand with independence. The shift from "nursing home" to "residential care facility" brought with it many changes designed to support independence. These include a room decorated with your personal possessions, privacy, help when needed, a limited kitchen, and—in many cases—freedom to manage your own schedule. This change has had a tremendous impact on the well-being of millions of people. I saw it firsthand with my parents, who spent the last eight years of their life together in a residential care facility in Fort Worth. In a later chapter, I will offer more detail on designing environments that can enhance your quality of live living with dementia.

Finding meaning in life. Part of our makeup as human beings is to seek meaning in what we do in life. Often what provides this meaning is feeling needed. The combination of being elderly and having Alzheimer's is likely to bring you lots of downtime. How do you plan to spend that time? Research on aging makes it clear that caring for others is a way of adding meaning that can really help. The "other" in this scenario does not have to be another person. A pet will do nicely, or even a plant. Reaching out to others remotely with a blog, as many people with dementia have done, is a great way to add meaning (even if, at the moment, you are not sure what "blog" means or how to create one).

In the book *Being Mortal: Medicine and What Matters in the End,* Atul Gawande tells the story of Bill Thomas, a physician, who took a job as medical director of a nursing home populated with disabled elderly residents, including many with Alzheimer's disease. He found the place depressing and lacking energy or spirit. Its passive, uninvolved residents seemed to be quietly waiting to die. Bill decided to shake things up. He added a dozen cats, dogs, hens, rabbits—and 100 canaries, one for each resident! Soon, many people had adopted a pet and each day were as concerned about its needs as their own.

Over the next two years, a team of researchers compared the results of these interventions with the residents to people living in a similar but traditional nursing home. They found that prescriptions dropped by half, costs dropped, and death rates declined. Variations of this result have been repeated many times in other studies. Today, many facilities use adaptations of this model. (I've been most impressed by the Sierra Vista facility here in Santa Fe.)

Becoming involved in the lives of animals, plants, family members, or children adds meaning to your life. In fact, almost anything that relates to reaching outside your own boundaries and self concerns to care for others can ignite a spark for living.

Look for opportunities in your own life to reach out and find meaningful connections.

Seeking Independence and Control

When you consider these four factors together, you can see they represent a common theme. Each of them is really about control over some aspect of your life, control that you could take for granted as a younger, more active person. Now that you are older and living with dementia, control becomes more and more precious every day. Living life to its fullest with dementia means fighting to maintain the personal integrity that comes with making choices, having friends, finding meaning by caring for others, and living in an environment that, to a large degree, you control.

You may struggle with the loss of some of your freedoms as your family tries to help but unwittingly compromises your independence. I remember my dad looking longingly at his car (a black Buick) each time he passed it on the way to dinner at the retirement home. Once he asked for the keys and, without comment, I joined him for a short drive around the parking lot, the first time he had driven since his stroke. Afterward he glowed with joy and pride. Despite doctor's orders, he loved his scotch, and our casual dinners in local restaurants turned into celebrations when the waiter brought that precious glass of Chivas Regal to the table.

Finding Meaning through Blogging

When you look around the world for people with Alzheimer's who stand out because of their independence and cognitive health, you find a remarkable group that is living longer, getting more satisfaction out of life, and finding ways to be engaged in living a complete life. As you read about these people on their blogs, it is hard not to be impressed with their positive attitude, despite the world's largely negative perspective on Alzheimer's.

Rick Phelps (phelps2645.blogspot.com), founder of Memory People, and Richard Taylor (richardtaylorphd.com), both well-known for their blogs, are just two examples of people who created public forums to chronicle their own experiences with the progression of dementia. I find their communications pretty amazing and recommend them to you, because I think they offer you a window of hope and understanding about what you will be experiencing in the future.

Here is Richard Taylor's advice on writing:

All of us who are the ingredients in the pressure cooker of Alzheimer's should write and share our thoughts and writings with others. E-mail them to family, whether or not they asked for them. Send them as letters to the editor. Send a couple of them to your newspaper for inclusion in its "area" edition.

All of us walking down Alzheimer's Avenue should write about our experiences in order to feel freer; in fact, we should feel a sense of obligation to share our day with others. It is good for us, the writers, and good for the readers.

What these two individuals with Alzheimer's show very clearly is that you, inside your own mind, most likely will be living a fully conscious, fully aware life. For some years to come, you may have the opportunity to experience many of the same kinds of joy you experience now. As you read these blogs, you can also see the courage and determination behind them. The authors speak to their own independence and insist on the fact that, inside, "I am still here." You can also see, as they reach out to share with others, how much meaning this sharing adds to their lives and how it strengthens them.

Using a Blog to Share What's on Your Mind

A blog today means that you are sharing these stories online. If this is what you choose to do, you, a friend, or family member can easily create a blog site for you with WordPress.com or a similar free site. You can also contribute to one of the existing blogs offered on the Dementia Action Alliance website (daanow. org) or Facebook.

You don't have to do this. If you can't imagine creating your own blog or using an existing blog because blogging is not part of your reality today, then let me reassure you. Think of a blog as any form of communication you create that shares your personal experience with dementia. Your "blog" can be written letters or stories. It can be based on conversations you have with caregivers about your experiences with dementia. Just creating some version of what you are experiencing and sharing it—in any form—will accomplish the same result.

Richard Taylor's well-known blog actually started just as an exercise for himself. Here is his description of why he started writing, from Alzheimer's Inside Out:

I don't write for others: I write for myself. I write to better understand myself, to remember my own insights, to work through my own issues, to find the right questions to ask, and to find a few new answers to give myself. I write to entertain myself and reassure myself that some of the old me is still there.

This sharing through your personal blog, whatever form it takes, adds health in many ways. It gives you a chance to show your independence, to connect socially with others, and to serve others (with or without Alzheimer's) through your messages. It exercises your consciousness so the drummers inside that connect the physical structure of the neurons in your brain with your experience play a real tune, one tied to meaning in your life, and resist degenerating into chaos. I think there is little doubt that sharing your experiences is one good path to a living a more active, joyful, full life.

KEY POINTS

- Research on aging suggests that the same four factors that make life worth living are common to almost everyone in both residential and home settings. These factors include:

Caring for others. It is important to find meaning in your life by living purposefully. Often this means caring for or giving to others. Caring for a pet can also serve this function.

Keeping your independence. It is essential to maintain a degree of independence and control over the important dimensions of your life. With dementia, you will have some dependence on others; however, every bit of independence you can find is precious.

Enjoying a social life. Enjoying a network of social connections with family and friends plus regular social contact is priceless and important to your physical and mental health.

Having a friendly environment. A friendly environment is one that supports your independence with an uncluttered, esthetic, functional design and has the best that today's technology can offer to entertain and provide reminders to support your daily habits.

- Reaching out with a blog or letters to communicate your feelings and experiences is a great way to share what is happening in your life, declare your independence, and strengthen your connections with others.

Ideas for your life? How might you act on them? What is the first step?

8

Building a Care Partner Team

Please know that caring for someone is not about your comfort but theirs. Remember you can give them great joy by sharing your thoughts, your love, and your stories with them, but I can't even begin to put into words what a gift you will receive back from them.

—Lori La Bey, *Alzheimer's Speaks* blog

Caregivers or care partners will take on many important roles in your Alzheimer's journey as guides, companions, nurses, and advocates. The quality of life you experience is likely to depend a great deal on them—on their energy, dedication, and willingness to embrace your reality. This chapter describes the approach to building a team of care partners. It also explains how technology will affect you and these care partners, today and in the future. Although the traditional terms "caregiver" and "caregiving" are used in most places throughout this book, I prefer to think of the people responsible for providing your care as equals or "care partners" and the service they provide as "caregiving."

Alzheimer's can place a huge burden on individual caregivers. In 2015, over 18.1 billion hours of caregiving (with an economic cost of $221.3 billion) were donated by individuals to family and friends with dementia in the United States. The typical length of care can range from four to 20 years! The caregivers' potential to become depressed increased by 56 percent, and many were also dealing with the high cost of providing care. Stress is also common for caregivers and the degree of stress is proportional to the degree of impairment you are experiencing as the partner with dementia. Other problems include hunger, anxiety, burnout, anger, sleeplessness, exhaustion, and social withdrawal. Health suffers because primary caregivers will often visit their doctors less often than normal and not pay attention to their own needs.

Your Care Partner Team

One-person caregiver models are one of the primary reasons for increased stress and health problems. Such models are not optimal for you or the caregiver. We need to look at other options. A team approach supported by technology is badly needed, so let's begin by building your care partner team.

What is the ideal composition of this team?

- The Team Leader is one of the primary care partners. The team leader may be the person who is physically present to provide most care, or a more technically oriented person who can serve as the coordinator.

- The Primary Care Partners can be one or several people who will be with you throughout the process.

- The Extended Team will be family and friends, nurses, professional caregivers, and others who will participate directly or indirectly in the caregiving process in different ways.

- The Virtual Team is made up of individuals who will provide caregiving support remotely, using a virtual caregiving system delivered through the Internet or other medium. Members of this team can be friends, volunteers from a dementia support group, or people who are part of a online caregiving network.

- The Robot Team or Computer-based Team may sound like fantasies at the moment, but much of the support provided by future caregivers will come from robots and computers combined with technology such as video monitors, GPS tools, and pattern recognition devices using artificial intelligence. Many countries currently have versions of caregiver robots in development.

There are three main reasons for building a team now, while you are still healthy:

1. By forming a team now, you will be creating a priceless resource that can help you later—and you retain some control over who is on the team.

2. By educating your team to "come to you" and follow the rules of your world while you are still healthy and can interact with them, you will establish patterns and open communication channels that will support you later. The sooner this happens, the better.

3. You set a very important precedent for later by relying on a team for support now. It is crucial to make clear from the beginning that you are not relying on a single person—like a spouse or child or other close family member—even if the primary caregiver will do most of the actual work.

For most members of your extended team and virtual team, who will have minor and non-labor-intensive roles, making a promise to be on your team is not a major commitment. It is providing an occasional hour or two a week at some time in the future. While this may not seem to be much now, when the time comes, it can make a huge difference to you and the primary caregivers. That hour will bring relief and respite, variety to counteract the boredom that can come with dementia, and dozens of long, joyful moments that will add quality to your life. Glenys Carl's book about her son Scott, *Hold My Hand: A Mother's Journey*, shows how powerful a network of caregivers can be, even with most contributing only a few hours.

Technology Can Help

To make an extended caregiving network successful, technology is required—not advanced technology, just today's technology focused on dementia. This technology makes remote caregiving feasible. It also offers advanced kinds of support to complement personal interactions, which may be compromised by repetitive behavior and by periods when not much is happening. Computers are infinitely patient and always vigilant, attributes that will serve you well, now and later.

Once your caregiver team is in place, giving them a basic education on the Caregiver Rules of the Road listed on Page xvii is essential. I also recommend that you choose one of the excellent books by professional caregivers, such as Jytte Lokvig's *Alzheimer's A to Z: A Quick-Reference Guide*, and give copies to your entire team. The rules for communication below come from her recent short book, *Alzheimer's and Dementia: Relationships and Teamwork Handbook*. While many of them may have limited relevance at the moment (since they were developed for people in the mid to late stages of dementia), sharing them with your caregivers will be a reminder of the importance of coming to you now and in the future. I have summarized them for convenience in the table below.

Rules for Communication

Listen: Individuals with moderate or advanced dementia may have difficulty forming words and sentences. When listening, "take a deep breath and concentrate on what he is trying to say and what his body language is telling you."

Avoid Baby Talk: No adult likes to be treated as if they had the mind of a child. Use normal speech.

Use Compliments and Humor: These pave the way for meaningful, joyful long moments.

Never Argue, Scold, or Criticize: All of these versions of "no" only serve to remind the person that you are evaluating their behavior against some standard in Earth-reality.

Avoid Saying, "Do You Remember?": Memory tests are not fair and disrupt healthy communication. It is important for you to "come to them," not pull them back to you.

Use "Do You Want?" with Care: Making concrete choices is good (Would you like an apple or a banana for lunch?). Abstract choices that involve concepts, or things that are not physically present, may cause confusion.

Avoid the Word "No": No is a powerful word that often has the opposite effect from what was intended. No can be confusing, because it may not be clear what behavior it relates to. It can also make the wrong behavior more likely; a golfer who tells himself not to hit the ball into the water hazard is actually telling the unconscious mind this is what to do!

Use Diversions and Loving Lies: This approach is valuable when logic and reasoning will not work and you need to communicate a message to change behavior quickly.

Respect Altered Realities: Remember that Earth-reality and Altzair-reality are not the same. Always respect the fact that what you are seeing and experiencing is not the view from Altzair.

Dealing with Caregivers

While some of these guidelines may not be relevant at this time, when you give them to your caregivers early, you send a strong message: "I need your help. I am a healthy adult with dementia. As time goes on, many of our traditional ways of communicating with each other will no longer work. Please use these guidelines and the Caregiver Rules of the Road to help our communications. Your willingness to do that will add many quality moments to my life. Thank you."

Dealing with your care partners is a complex dance. "No, I am not a child." "Yes, please speak to me as an adult but use clear, concrete language." "No, don't take over management of my finances." "Yes, I need your help." "No, I don't understand." "Yes, listen to me, not to my words." On the one hand, you are looking inside and cherishing your independence, while in the dance, the other hand is constantly extended to your partners. You are seeking their help and support—but not unlimited support; just the amount you need.

Greg O'Brien describes this dance well:

Caregivers and individuals living with the diagnosis both travel down the same Alzheimer's Boulevard; however, my lane has some different potholes than my wife's, and vice versa.

We each are forced to make different detours. Sometimes we can walk hand in hand and other times we are miles apart. We label the trip with the same name but we are on two different journeys.

Taking Extra Time Is OK

Being slow in your responses, acting confused for a few moments, not finding the right word in a conversation, or not recalling the name of a close relative—all of these can lead to a very common reaction. Your caregivers want to help by filling in the blanks with the right word, but many times, this is not the help you wanted. You didn't mind not having the answer immediately or working through your confusion; in fact, if possible, you wanted to figure things out on your own. Let your caregivers know that these pauses and delays are part of you now. From your perspective, there is no need to rush to fill in the blanks. Ambiguity is OK. You live with it all of the time.

How do you want others to treat the person that is you with dementia? It may not be clear. You are an adult, not a child, so you don't want to be treated as a child. But you are a different adult now, so while you want others to respect your independence, at times you will also need help and support. The person that is you is a moving target that changes to some degree each day. You want your caregivers to recognize these changes and keep up with the target. You want them to be paying attention and to keep the dialogue going.

This excerpt from Richard Taylor's presentation at the 2014 Alzheimer's Disease International Conference speaks to these changing needs:

A Message to My Family

Now (a month after diagnosis) is a time to have a meeting of the family minds and hearts.

The burden of change is more on others than on persons living with dementia.

Our needs do not lessen, nor are they reduced in number as the number and severity of our symptoms increase.

We were, are, and will be up to about two minutes after we draw our last breath whole human beings.

We need enablers, not disablers. Sometimes we need re-ablers.

We need support to stay into today.

KEY POINTS

- Your caregivers or care partners will take on many important roles in your Alzheimer's journey, as guides, companions, nurses, and advocates.

- The term "care partner" is used in many places to remind you that you are an active participant in the process of working with a caregiver to live a full life.

- The traditional, one-person caregiver model is not healthy for you or the caregiver. You need a team. Your team will consist of:

Team Leader

Primary Care Partners

Extended Care Partners

Virtual Care Partners

Robot or Computer-based Partners

- The team leader will use today's technology for communication, scheduling, and coordinating the activities of the team.

- Encourage your team to use the Rules for Communication in this chapter and the Care Partner Rules of the Road to support their interactions with you and preserve the integrity of your personhood.

- In the dance of dementia, your caregivers will need to learn their roles and to respect yours as an independent, adult being seeking just the help you need, not unlimited support.

Ideas for your life? How might you act on them? What is the first step?

9

Planning Now to Secure Your Future

Passing the baton has significance on many fronts—on a track, at home, at work, in disease and into eternity. In the relay race of life, one cannot run alone. You sprint your leg as best possible, then hand off with precision, letting others carry you as they can.
—Greg O'Brien, *On Pluto: Inside the Mind of Alzheimer's*

One of the most unforgiving aspects of Alzheimer's is that the disease may eventually affect your speech. Stroke patients often experience similar difficulties. You are likely to be thinking or knowing things that you would like to express but find it difficult at times to do so. What this means practically is that the clock is ticking.

In the next few weeks or months, you need to do the planning that will create the foundation for a full and joyful life—and you don't have any time to waste. This is one area where everyone in the Alzheimer's community—individuals, physicians, families, professional caregivers, attorneys, and financial planners—seems to agree! Let's get to work.

Four Key Areas to Consider

Financial Planning

Decisions about wills, estates, trusts, and how your family will manage the costs of care in the late stages, are all important topics to address now, while you are judged to be mentally competent. The most important legal document to consider is the durable *power of attorney*. This document authorizes a trusted family member, friend, or advisor to act as your agent in a variety of financial and legal matters. You can set this up to be effective immediately, or at some point in the future based on a specific event; for example, if you are moved to a residential care facility.

Healthcare Directives

These documents are crucial for defining the kinds of care that you do and do not want to receive later in life when you can no longer speak for yourself. They include:

A living will. Typically, this document provides specific instructions about the course of treatment and the limits of treatment. It may include information on whether or not you want special services such as pain relief, resuscitation, tube feeding, the use of ventilators, and the use of antibiotics. Medicine today is designed to save and extend life with no boundaries on the pain or inconvenience to the patient. Your living will provides crucial directives that express your wishes when you are not capable of doing so.

A healthcare proxy. This is a legal document that allows you to appoint someone you trust to make healthcare decisions for you when you are unable, for any reason, to make these decisions for yourself. Because everyone with Alzheimer's will need a proxy at some point, it is important to select one now. Close family members such as a spouse or child don't always make the best proxies because of their emotional involvement. Select someone you trust who will be likely to make good, objective decisions at a time when there may be confusion, high emotions, and perhaps some pressure from family members.

Hospice care. This important end-of-life option is not readily available for people with Alzheimer's. To trigger hospice care, an individual has to meet the requirements of mental competence, which cannot be met in the later stages. Hospice provides medical services, emotional and spiritual support, and help for family members, all with a focus on keeping you comfortable and improving the quality of your life. *I recommend that you create your own hospice directive and include it in your living will. Every person with Alzheimer's needs hospice care at the end of life.* See the sample hospice care agreement for Alzheimer's in my book, *The Long Moment: Communicating with the Alzheimer's Mind.*

Decisions about Care and Where You Will Live

Your choices now will help to guide the decisions that your family and other caregivers will need to make at a later time.

Who will be part of your caregiver team? This topic was covered in the previous chapter. As you know, it is very important to the quality of your life to recruit the members of this team now and begin to train them to support you.

At some time in the future, living with Alzheimer's, you will probably need a good deal of support. Where would you like to live? Do you have the option to live at home with a supportive care giver network to help, or will the services of a special memory-care facility be needed? Discussing these topics now will help to guide the best decisions later, even if the answers to these questions are not 100 percent clear at the moment.

Life Quality Choices

These important decisions made early in the process help set up the optimal conditions you will need later to support a complete and joyful life. I think the best approach is to take out a tablet and, alone or with close family or caregivers present, write out the answers to the following questions:

- What are the everyday things that you enjoy most or that bring the most quality to your life?

- What could friends and family do to add joy and quality to your life? Do you want them to visit, write letters, send photos? What would be most meaningful for you?

- If you have a bucket list, it may have some big things you would like to do. Is there anything else you might consider adding to this list?

- What are your favorite places?

- What are the activities or hobbies that you enjoy the most, the ones that help to make life worth living?

- What are the anchors that connect you with your personal history? Pictures? Videos? Stories? Music? Knowing your preferences will help your caregivers add joyful moments later.

Make a Video

The documents described above serve as concise but powerful directives to your family, physicians, caregivers, and others. They explain in detail your choices about your future care. That's the good news. The bad news is that when the time comes to use them, they may be almost worthless.

It can be difficult for family or physicians to make tough decisions about your care in a highly charged emotional setting, based on a few words you wrote years before. As Atul Gawande says in his book, *Being Mortal: Medicine and What Matters in the End*, the traditional healthcare directives described above are often not sufficient, given the conflicting pressures around complex medical decisions made by family near the end of life.

His recommendation, which I agree with completely, is that once the key documents above are ready, you sit down with your family and go over each of your choices on video, so that everyone involved can see what you are thinking and feeling about these decisions. The video then becomes the record to keep, to remind everyone exactly what you wanted—in your own words.

Use a Checklist

Situations that involve aging, disease, multiple family members, and legal documents can be difficult to resolve. They are also prone to errors and mistakes. You are currently in one of these situations (as if you had not already figured that out). To make the best of it, you will need the help of a team and a personal video to communicate your wishes. To cut through the noise and potential for information overload, you will also need a checklist. A simple checklist reminds everyone involved what has been done and what still needs to be done. I have included a sample list at the end of the chapter. Get on it!

There is some urgency to do the vital planning in these four areas now, while no one is questioning your capability, since this planning is one of the keys to retaining a measure of independence and control over the quality of the rest of your life.

My Planning Checklist

___1. My will and related legal documents

___2. My power of attorney

___3. My healthcare directives
  - Living will
  - Healthcare proxy
  - Hospice choices
  - Video describing all choices

___4. Options for places where I will live

___5. My financial plan

___6. My life quality choices
  - Friends and family
  - Favorite places
  - Bucket list
  - Favorite activities
  - Personal anchors

___7. My care partner team

___8. Memory support tools
  - Reminisce cards (pictures of my life history)
  - Communication cards (things I want to say)
  - List of favorite music
  - List of favorite movies

KEY POINTS

- It is important to do the planning needed to secure your future as soon as possible. There are four key areas to consider:

  Financial planning. Key topics include decisions about wills, estates, cost of your care in the late stages, and—most important—creating a durable power of attorney.

  Healthcare directives. Key documents include a living will, a healthcare proxy, and a personal hospice guide (since you will not be eligible for traditional hospice care later).

  Caregiver/living choices. These are decisions about your care partner team and where you choose to live based on the available options.

  Life quality choices. To live a full life with dementia, it is essential for you and your care partners to understand what things define a quality life for you. Creating a bucket list, building a personal history, connecting with key family members or friends, selecting hobbies or other activities of interest—all represent ways to define what life quality means to you.

- Make a short video of yourself describing briefly each of your decisions above: financial choices, health directive choices, and quality of life choices. It will have much more weight than words in a document or opinions of family members at a later time when your intentions may no longer be clear.

- Checklist: Use the simple checklist included in this chapter to keep track of all the documents and video you need to prepare.

Ideas for your life? How might you act on them? What is the first step?

10

Physical and Mental Activities to Support a Good Life

If you can't take classes or go out dancing four times a week, then dance as much as you can. More is better. And do it now, the sooner the better. It's essential to start building your cognitive reserve now. Some day you'll need as many of those stepping-stones across the creek as possible. Don't wait—start building them now.

—Richard Powers
From a *CCAL* blog post titled "Dancing Makes You Smarter"

Taking control of your life with dementia means, in part, doing the obvious things that research plus the experiences of others with dementia have demonstrated will make a difference. This chapter outlines some of these important, established behaviors that I recommend. Your goal is to claim some of the latent capacities that can potentially move your brain in the direction of Resilient Aging and slow the onset of dementia symptoms. From my perspective, these are the low-hanging fruit on the brain's tree of life that most people can enjoy.

Meditation

The practice of meditation can have a profound effect on the health of the brain in ways that seem to reduce the symptoms of Alzheimer's. Meditation can be either religious or non-religious in nature. What distinguishes it from other activities is the act of letting go of the normal chatter in the mind. This release is often accomplished by focusing on a single thing such as an object, a sound, a word, or simply the breath. Typically, a person in meditation is experiencing a subtle shift in awareness; they are aware of the world but somewhat detached from it.

Meditation stimulates and exercises specific areas of your brain. Think of these areas as "muscles" that are underdeveloped. Using them regularly may help give your mind some of the properties associated with Resilient Aging that support normal cognitive functioning.

Research also shows that meditation reduces stress, increases happiness and harmony, improves sleep, and enhances your overall sense of well-being. Most important, it reduces your chances of becoming depressed. This last point is significant because, as I described in Chapter 2, many people living with dementia battle depression, especially in the early stages.

I think the easiest way to add meditation to your daily routine is to purchase a CD or one of the many meditation apps available, select a meditation you enjoy, and then listen to it every day. Having a recorded guide will help you deal with distractions and create a practice you can follow regularly.

One item from the benefits listed above is worth repeating if getting to sleep is a problem for you. Because meditation can calm some of the chatter and ruminations in your mind, *it can be very helpful as a sleep aid.*

Singing

The act of singing is a powerful, healthy stimulant for your mind, heart, and body. It combines sound, words, music, emotions, and breathing in a way that can be exciting, relaxing, or joyful. Every marching army in history has had its own collection of songs, because taking the song from inside you and projecting it into the world is a way of releasing fear. Singing quiets the mind and ripples across all of your senses, often bringing emotions to the surface. Whether you do it alone, in a group, or with your caregivers, I think you will be pleasantly surprised at the benefits of adding singing to your daily routine.

Physical Exercise

Research has established a strong connection between physical health and exercise—and your physical health affects your mental health—so I encourage you to have a daily exercise routine, even if this involves little more than walking. Especially valuable for your brain is any physical routine that forces you to move in patterns. Dancing, swimming, tai chi, qigong, yoga, and the many modern variations of aerobics are some of the best ways to exercise.

Mental Stimulation

There is a strong association between actively using your brain and delaying the onset of dementia symptoms. Research confirms that this remains true for individuals in the early stages of Alzheimer's. *Use it or lose it* is a good warning to heed. Games such as bridge, Scrabble, or backgammon, and mental puzzles of any kind (crosswords, Sudoku, math problems, completion exercises) all may help. Reading and listening to books, writing letters and e-mails, keeping a journal, or doing any of the many other things that exercise the verbal, reasoning side of your mind may increase your brain's resiliency in the face of dementia. Researchers have identified two of the above activities as especially effective in delaying the onset of dementia symptoms—reading and crossword puzzles—so have fun!

Relaxation

When my spouse Marilyn is chilling out for a day of relaxation, I will tease her about being in a "la la zone," a place that is very healthy because she is letting go and detaching from worries about finances, clients, housework—or tending to me (unfortunately). Finding a way to reduce stress, frustration, haste, judgment, and other negative feelings that interfere with your joy can be very helpful. Your target is simply to interpret what is happening around you with a light touch and good humor, so that it doesn't add to your stress. Low stress supports good mental health and increased cognitive resiliency.

Finding Security

Security supports your mental health by reducing worry and eliminating many of the daily "battles" that you fight to get along. Physical security and safety, along with financial, emotional, and environmental security, are all aspects of your life that will reward your attention. You may not, at this time, have good control over all of these things, but doing what you can now to plan for a future where they are well-managed will support your current and future health.

Adjusting Your Attitude

There are no surprises here. Much of this book offers choices and information that support a positive, open-minded attitude toward living life. Chapters on choosing to live life to its fullest, adding happy or positive moments every day, embracing your life history, using affirmations, and improving communication offer ideas and help on this topic.

Sleep

As I described in Chapter 5, longer and deeper sleep means more effective flushing of unwanted materials (including peptides associated with Alzheimer's) from the brain. While I cannot guarantee that it will help delay or slow the onset of your dementia, the potential here is too great to ignore. Find a way, with or without pills, to sleep well. Is sleeping well one key to resilient aging? It is too early to know definitively, but as a gambling man, I would say it is a good possibility.

Dancing

I confess, I have saved the best for last. Dancing deserves some special recognition here. In a major research study on the specific activities of people over 75 that delayed the onset of dementia, *dancing was the star*. People who danced regularly saw a 76 percent reduction in the risk of dementia! There are many things to like here: pattern-oriented movements, the connection to music, and, not least, working with a partner to be aware of and responsive to their actions. What is special about dancing that distinguishes it from mental activities such as crossword puzzles (which delay the onset of symptoms temporarily) is that the benefits will persist throughout your life with Alzheimer's.

Resilient Aging

Remember the group of nuns who had Alzheimer's but showed few or no symptoms and the concept of Resilient Aging? This is a very important concept for anyone with dementia, because it suggests that, under the right conditions, the symptoms of dementia can be reduced significantly. As you review the above list of physical and mental activities that support living a normal life, you will see that most, if not all, fit the lifestyles of the nuns in this study!

KEY POINTS

- One approach for taking control of your life with dementia is to engage in the physical and mental activities that support *Resilient Aging*.

- Resilient Aging is a concept that explains why some brains age in a manner that is healthier and more likely to preserve normal cognitive functionality.

- While there is no guarantee that acting to promote Resilient Aging will reduce your dementia symptoms or delay the onset of dementia, there is some possible benefit here.

- Activities that may support Resilient Aging include:

  Meditation
  Singing
  Exercise
  Mental stimulation
  Relaxation
  Having a secure, low-stress environment
  Positive attitude
  Sleep
  Dancing

- Notice that the population of nuns described in Chapter 4 who had Alzheimer's but showed few or none of the symptoms engage in most of the above list of activities on a regular basis!

Ideas for your life? How might you act on them? What is the first step?

11

Defining Your Personal Anchors

Mom's residential facility has a locked Alzheimer's unit to keep residents from wandering and harming themselves. One evening after dinner I was sitting with mom quietly watching TV when the door to the locked unit opened as an aide escorted two gentlemen to a nearby, small conference room. As they approached, one of the men turned to me and said, "We will be having a Board meeting, discussing business and then headed for a boys' night out." As I watched, the aide seated both men at the table, handed them newspapers, pencils and paper then closed the door! What a great way to acknowledge that both of these gentlemen had a history as productive businessmen and while dementia had taken some of that away, at their core they were still the same people, anchored to their past experiences.

—Katherine Frazier, from stories about her mother,

Emilou, at a residential treatment facility in Florida

In Chapter 8, I described a number of specific ways that your friends and caregivers can support the integrity of your personhood through their behavior and their attitudes toward dementia. Not surprisingly, you also play a major role in this process. There are several key things you can do that may provide strong anchors for your individual well-being throughout the Alzheimer's process.

To begin, I want you to think for a moment about what makes you a "person" based on a common sense definition of this term. (Note that typically we think of *both* children and adults as complete persons; children quickly become full "persons" at a very young age.) You are a person because you have a unique identity, a unique set of life experiences, and a unique personality. All of these things (and more) rolled up together define you and quickly separate you from every other being on the planet.

Until now, your integrity as a person has probably never been threatened or challenged. It is as much a part of you as ham in a ham-and-egg sandwich. Alzheimer's, however, can create some confusion here. On the surface, your family and others will see the handicaps the disease creates for you, and in these changes may also see a different *you*. Unfortunately, this can occur without their understanding that the underlying person that is you has not changed. You will always be the same unique, independent being with your own personality, but dementia can mask this being with the noise and interruptions it brings. It may also prevent you from expressing your independence or personhood so others can relate to it.

How Others Can Help Define You

Part of the problem comes from a misunderstanding. While it's true that your personhood is about you—your identity, your personality, your interests and needs—it's also true that you don't exist in isolation. Much of your personality is actually defined by others and how you relate to them. These *others* can be family, organizations, employers, or any type of social entity.

From a broad perspective, it is these relationships that help to fully define who you are.

Your personal history is filled with the anchors needed to ground you and those around you in the reality of "who you are" and "how others can relate to you." Let me give you a quick example. Imagine that your family is visiting today and that in the group is a grandson and a granddaughter. They don't have any real idea what your Alzheimer's diagnosis means or what to expect because of it. In fact, it doesn't matter. When they visit, it is your role in their life—grandparent—that matters and will always dominate their perception of you. This is the anchor they will use to guide their interactions with you. You will always be their grandparent.

Similar anchors can be found with all your friends, family, and caregivers, now and in the future. Your identity as a person is defined in part by how you relate to other people through the different roles that are part of your life. These roles—grandparent, spouse, partner, and many more—bring relevance and realness to your interactions with others even when you have lost your voice.

The Importance of Sharing Your Personal History

Let's look at another quick example. It is five years from now and dementia may have diminished your ability to speak what is on your mind and to function every day without support. One of your caregivers is a professional nurse who sees many people daily in her caregiving role. There are two ways she can relate to you:

1. You are simply another patient with a certain set of needs that require care.

2. You are Andy Jackson, a former math teacher from Ohio, married with two adult children, a former golfer, and active supporter of the Sierra Club.

Shared knowledge of your personal history changes things. The more shared knowledge, the easier it is for your personhood to shine through the noise of dementia. Each of the various roles in life that you have played is a social lifeline that connects you and other people solidly with an identity that they can relate to. Being seen as a grandparent or partner or banker or golfer forges a stronger, more personal connection than "patient."

What are these anchors or roles that connect you and others with your personhood? Borrowing from the excellent work of Barbara Conforti at York College, I'll divide them into three categories: identity, purpose, and belonging.

Personal Anchors

1. Identity
Anchors that help to identify how you relate to others in your life:
- Parent
- Child
- Spouse
- Friend
- Partner

2. Purpose
Anchors that reflect roles tied to a sense of purpose or goals:
- Career (artist, accountant, lawyer, etc.)
- Mentor
- Student
- Manager/director/leader
- Volunteer

3. Belonging

Anchors that describe your role as a member of groups or organizations:

- Owner
- Fan
- Neighbor
- Participant

A big part of personhood is your life story. Much of this story is already written and will stay with you throughout the Alzheimer's process. Many of the chapters in this story will be connected through the roles outlined above. Being a grandfather or spouse, for example, immediately adds richness and history to your interactions with others and connects you across the boundaries of the past, present, and future.

Living fully also means embracing the context that each of these roles creates for you. You may not remember the name of a high school tennis coach or the cousin whom you vacationed with in Alaska, but you will always remember how to play tennis and the beauty of the mountains surrounding Juneau.

When you construct your personal history, items tied to these anchors—pictures, videos, stories—are especially important because they will never lose their meaning. Each of these anchors is also a reminder to others of your completeness as an independent, adult person. Finally, each offers a specific way of connecting with you that enhances meaningful communications and expands your chance for more and longer joyful moments.

KEY POINTS

- You are a person because you have a unique identity, a unique set of life experiences, and a unique personality.

- Until now, your integrity as a person has probably never been threatened or challenged. Dementia may change this because family and friends may have trouble seeing you through the stigma and confusion it can create.

- One thing that can help here is to use the relationships you have with other people and organizations to anchor your identity in ways that make it clear *who you are as a person.*

- These relationships are an important part of your personal history that will stay with you throughout your Alzheimer's journey.

- There are three types of personal anchors that connect you with others:

  Identity: Anchors that help to identify how you relate to others in your life (parent, child, spouse).

  Purpose: Anchors that represent roles tied to goals, employment, or a sense of purpose (teacher, student, manager).

  Belonging: Anchors that describe your role as a member of groups or organizations (volunteer, leader, owner).

- Living fully with dementia means embracing these important anchors connecting you with others. They are part of your personal history throughout your journey and can add many positive moments to your life.

Ideas for your life? How might you act on them? What is the first step?

12

Saving Your Personal History in a Companion Mind

You could say that yes, the Internet is making us stupider, or you could say that we're just using Google and other search engines as an extension of our brains. Experts call this "transactive memory." Basically, you remember where to get the information—just not the information itself. The concept of transactive memory is nothing new: prior to the digital age, we used non-digital "experts"—friends or books. The search engine has just made that process a whole lot easier.

"Our brains rely on the Internet for memory in much the same way they rely on the memory of a friend, family member, or co-worker," Betsy Sparrow of Harvard, explains. "We remember less through knowing information itself than by knowing where the information can be found."
—Ed Oswald, PC World

This chapter is part reality and part fiction but as you read these words, the fiction part is quickly becoming reality—and over the next three years, much of it will *be* reality, a reality that can have a very significant impact on the quality of your life with dementia.

The Best Companion

Let's begin with a question. Imagine for a moment that you did not need to make the Alzheimer's journey alone but were permitted to have a companion and that your choice is unlimited. You can choose any companion that you want. Who would you select? Your spouse? Your best friend? Another family member? An Alzheimer's professional? Who will make the best companion?

You know, of course, based on the title of this chapter, that I am setting you up. The obvious choice, if it were possible, would be the healthy, pre-dementia version of you! Who better to understand your personal history, your challenges and feelings about Alzheimer's, your everyday needs and habits, or your likes and dislikes? There is no one else who can come close to *you* in understanding *your* reality.

But of course, this is not possible. You cannot be in two places at once—living with dementia and at the same time joining yourself as an ally with your full pre-dementia consciousness. Correct? Perhaps in a movie, this is possible. A machine is invented that somehow creates a duplicate of your mind, freezes it, and then saves it for later use. We do this now with embryos that are frozen until needed, then fertilized and implanted in a donor's uterus to create a baby. We also replace the functions of diseased organs using stem cells, which can replicate most organs in the body. Could there be a way to do this with your mind?

Believe it or not, the answer is a resounding "yes." If we think digitally instead of biologically, we have the technology available today to save much of the content of your mind, your history, and your experiences living in Earth-reality and give it back to you to use throughout the Alzheimer's journey!

A Companion Mind

This chapter introduces the concept of a "companion mind." What does this mean? A companion mind is simply a digital version of part of your healthy, pre-dementia mind. Memories, thoughts, images, feelings, behaviors—all have some form of digital representation. This is the ally we have been seeking that offers the most hope for you on the Alzheimer's journey because as a companion, it has no equal. This digital mind represents a limited but very powerful version of you, your memories, your behaviors, your experiences—before the onset of dementia.

This brings us back to an important question: "Is this fantasy or reality? Is it possible to create a replica of your current mind that becomes a companion on your journey with dementia?" The answer may surprise you. Not only is it possible, the process for doing this has existed for many years and billions of people globally have already created limited versions of companion minds that they use daily!

The Content of Social Media

Think for a moment about a social media account such as you might find on Facebook or LinkedIn. What does it contain? Quite a lot, actually. It has a limited version of your personal history. It knows your friends and family, and connects with their history. It tracks what you and your friends are doing now. It understands your preferences, your likes and dislikes—and your feelings about many issues. Based on your behavior, it connects you with many people and events in which it predicts you might have an interest. In short, it does a pretty good job of digitally creating a reality that represents some parts of your consciousness.

Social media accounts, search engines, blogs, advertising engines, and other Internet programs offer something else that is very important in our search for the best companion for your dementia journey. Because these are digital tools, the personal history and memories they depend on are grounded in very concrete things such as photos, videos, stories, recordings, letters, notes, or familiar places. And all of these things are anchored to a "timeline" and a calendar.

Now you can see where I am headed with this chapter. With a little work, using technology that already exists and is user-friendly, you can construct a companion mind today that will serve you in many ways during your life with dementia. It is that simple. While we think that much of the technology that I describe above is really designed for teenagers (which is true), it is also available to you and with some recent developments I will describe later, becoming more available every day.

Acting Now to Benefit Later

At the start of this chapter, I mentioned the idea of "freezing your mind" and saving it for later use. While that concept probably is fantasy, a more limited version of it is not. You *can* preserve much of the content of your mind now, using available tools for storing digital information, and have access to this information later, throughout your life with dementia. There are some things you can do with this intelligence now, such as recognizing the important people in your life, generating prompts to help manage everyday habits, communicating with family and others—so there is some immediate value. But a tsunami of applications and the technology to support them are currently being developed that will soon (in the next few years) transform this stored data into a true companion mind, a mind so powerful and useful that every person with dementia globally will want one. I think the existence of this digital mind will also change the mechanics of person-centered dementia care forever.

There is an important catch here. We don't know the full details yet about how you can best use a companion mind to add quality to your life of living with dementia. The intelligence stored in the mind and the related apps have to work for you, not the inventors, and your world is not always accessible. The range of answers here can go from "you will get some modest benefit" to "this changes everything and will have a major impact on the quality of your life." While I lean toward the latter answer, there is still much work to be done to demonstrate that it is correct. This idea is a bit of a gamble. The catch is *you cannot wait.* If you don't save your personal history digitally now, while you are still healthy, you will not have access to this history later, when you need it, during your Alzheimer's journey.

My strong recommendation is that you and your care partners get to work, collecting information about your personal history and other details of your pre-dementia life, store it digitally, and construct the core of a companion mind that can serve you later.

Building Your Companion Mind

A companion mind, in essence, has just two components: 1) the information about your personal history that is stored in the mind and, 2) all of the applications that connect to the mind and use this history for your benefit. Since you are probably not a computer nerd, the idea of storing your history digitally may seem like a daunting task. Actually, as you will see, because of the programs available today, with the help of your caregiver team, it will be fairly simple. Collecting the information, however, may be more of a challenge because it is likely to come from many sources. Let me walk you through the process.

Step 1: Collect the Information You Want to Include

The information you want to use can come from you and from family members, friends, and organizations that share part of your history. It may include:

- Pictures or videos of yourself, family, friends, colleagues, and others that are meaningful to you.

- Pictures or videos of significant places, activities, or events in your life such as schools or colleges, your wedding, your job, hobbies, a church, or a favorite museum or park.

- Letters or audio/video recordings from friends and family reminding you of parts of your history and offering support, humor, stories, or anything else appropriate.

- A list of your favorite books, music, poems, movies, and possibly recordings or digital versions of these. Several companies offer packaged collections of music you might like.

- Information about your caregiver team. Who is on the team? Where do they live? What are their roles? How do you connect to them to communicate?

- A collection of your favorite jokes or cartoons.

- A timeline or chart connecting the important events in your life so you can quickly see where you were living and what you were doing at any time.

In addition to this personal history, your companion mind will also store information about your life today, including a daily schedule, daily routines or habits, your physical location, people you are in contact with, typical communications, and typical problems or needs.

If you are a regular user of Facebook or any of the other major social networking sites, the above list would be quite familiar except for some of the historical data. These sites do an excellent job of blending your personal history and your current schedule and activities with a timeline, if you willing to share all of this with your care partners.

Step 2: Storing Your Personal History in a Digital Format or Companion Mind

This is actually a pretty straightforward process because creating the content of your personal history also means that you have saved it for later use. Many devices today actually create digital versions of the items listed above and store them automatically in an appropriate format. A smartphone, for example, can take photos, videos, and recordings; copy documents; save and play music; and much more. Most computers today have software with similar functionality. Once an item is stored, you can then send it to any location to be saved and integrated into your companion mind.

What is still missing—but coming quickly—is the dedicated "mind" program designed specifically to save and organize your personal history, integrate it with your daily activities now, and provide a set of tools or apps focused on dementia. Programs that I will describe below such as MindPartner, Mind-Mate, WindowMirror, and others have some of these features.

Social networking sites such as Facebook, Google+, LinkedIn, and others also have useful features but are not suitable as a basis for your companion mind. As I said in the beginning, it is worthwhile to save your personal history now even though the companion mind product and apps to use it are still being developed.

Step 3: Use Your Companion Mind Apps to Add Quality to Your Life

Now we get to the fun part. The beauty of having your personal history stored in a digital format is that *it can be made accessible to you whenever and wherever you need it*. How will you use it? You will be able to do this through many different tools and applications, a few of which are currently available while many more are in development now. As you will see, the uses are potentially unlimited: to support short-term memory loss (perhaps the most important use); to communicate; to entertain; to add joy and other positive emotions; to connect with your caregivers; to help with everyday habits; and much more.

Benefitting from a companion mind is that simple. Build it using items from your personal history plus daily activities, and then use it throughout the Alzheimer's journey as needed, most likely through a special set of tools or apps. Since many of the components of this partner mind will be dealing with issues that relate to short-term memory loss, it will be helpful to understand more about this aspect so you will know what to expect.

Apps to Support Short-term Memory

Short-term memory refers to remembering the things you did in the last few minutes or hours. If you cannot remember what you had for breakfast this morning, or why you came into the kitchen a few minutes ago, these are problems with short-term memory.

Alzheimer's disease has the most impact on short-term memory because recent events are not well-anchored in the mind. The technical term is *consolidation*. Until a memory is consolidated, it isn't organized and stored in a manner that allows it to become a permanent part of your mind. Think of recent events as being located in a temporary place, in a sort of holding pattern, until some of them eventually become permanent memories.

As Alzheimer's destroys brain cells, it can create havoc with short-term memory, making it difficult to recall what happened recently. It also can disrupt the connections between your long-term memories and what is happening now. You won't forget your spouse or close friends (in the early to middle stages of dementia), but you may be confused by their presence or behavior in the short term. This can be frustrating for both you and them, and can have a negative impact on what you are experiencing in the moment.

How a Sample App Might Work

How do we fix this? We don't. We can't until the magic pill to cure Alzheimer's becomes available. Your job in the meantime is to find a way to turn these negative moments into moments that are positive or at least neutral—and this is where a companion mind can help. To illustrate how this process might work, we will invent a simple tool called the "Friends and Family App." How does it work?

Whenever a friend or family member enters your home, the app recognizes them and announces their presence to you ("Aunt Mary is in the house"). In this example, your companion mind, through the app, has helped you connect the person with their name and their presence in the house—all things you possibly know, but that may be confusing because of problems with short-term memory. By reducing the potential for confusion, it takes a moment that might be negative because of your uncertainty and gives it a chance to be positive or at least neutral.

Does this sound like a fantasy? Well, it's not! A recent app developed by Samsung, Backup Memory, actually works exactly this way, and several similar apps are currently being tested. Forgetting the names of family and friends is a common part of aging made worse by dementia. The Samsung app uses a smartphone that you keep in a pocket or purse. As long as the friend or family member visiting has a mobile device with the same app, it will announce their presence! You can find this app in the Google Play store for free.

Many other companies have products and apps available now that can help. While not designed specifically for people with dementia, Amazon's Echo (amazon.com/echo), a portable speaker coupled with a smart personal assistant, offers a variety of helpful tools now, such as answering questions, taking instructions ("I want to watch TV"), or entertaining you by playing music or reading you a book.

WindowMirror (windowmirror.com) is startup company with another smart product that offers many features, including a "repeat" feature that plays back the last 60 seconds of a conversation to help you keep track. MindMate (mindmate-app.com), a product that is popular in the UK, contains applications for you as well as your family and people in residential care facilities. It has apps for games and everyday reminders, and can store the highlights of your personal history.

Finally and not least, there are my own apps, available as part of the MindPartner (mindpartner.org) program. These include an app for smartphones or tablets to support communication by allowing you to quickly select from a set of standard or custom messages to share a thought with your family or friends. Another app saves parts of your history in a set of "Reminisce cards" and then gives it back to you for stimulation or entertainment. All of these companies and their products use the concept of a companion mind to support you in different ways.

Other Roles for Your Companion Mind

Your companion mind isn't designed just to help with simple tasks like recognizing a friend. It can help with communication by replacing speech with other ways of sharing what you want to say, such as cards or images. It can support your happiness by feeding you pictures or stories or music from your personal history that you consider to be joyful. It can alleviate some of the frustration that comes from not remembering why you are in the kitchen or bathroom with simple reminders or prompts linked to a daily activity schedule. The options are almost unlimited.

What's the overall goal here? Giving yourself access to your personal history, by using a companion mind plus apps that support this history, offers you the opportunity to add many positive long moments to your life in the next few years. The next step here, beyond saving your personal history, is to capture other parts of your experience such as cognitive functions, emotions, preferences, and behaviors that are a normal part of your life before dementia. A true companion mind might then use this enhanced intelligence to program a personal assistant or other applications to provide very smart, very personal kinds of support—as you might expect from a family member. You can see a proposed list of apps associated with my product, MindPartner, in Appendix A.

Remember that a companion mind is not a mysterious, abstract concept that depends on robots and artificial intelligence (although in the future, these may be valuable components). Rather, it is simply a digital version of your personal history organized so that it is accessible when needed. Because your companion mind works to keep you in touch with this history, it becomes a powerful ally in your quest to live a full life. Building your companion mind now, while you can, is a wise investment even though the full power of the technology and related applications needed to support it, and your life with dementia, will not be available for several years. You will want to take advantage of this technology and the help that it offers as soon as possible.

This chapter completes the set of things you might do to prepare yourself for the Alzheimer's journey. The next section of the book offers a collection of practical tools and ideas to support the concept of living life to its fullest with dementia.

KEY POINTS

- While many of your long-term memories and personal history will remain intact throughout your Alzheimer's journey, they may not be accessible, in the moment, because of short-term memory loss.

- Short-term memory loss means that recent events, experienced in the past few minutes or hours, are often lost because your mind cannot consolidate these experiences into memories and save them for later use.

- A "companion mind" that contains a digital summary of your personal history, your preferences, and your experiences might help. It would be available 24/7, as needed, to provide memories and information that can add joy and quality to your life.

- You and your caregiver team will construct this companion mind using the simple online tools that are available today for storing pictures, videos, music, and other information.

- Storing these data in a companion mind is just the first step. Once you have saved your personal history, current activities, and preferences in a digital format, developers will then be able to access this history to create tools called "apps" that are designed to help you live a full life.

- For example, you may have trouble remembering names of friends and family members. One app will help recognize their faces and remind you of their names. Another version of this app sees the location of the person relative to you and announces when they visit your room or home.

Ideas for your life? How might you act on them? What is the first step?

LIVING A FULL LIFE WITH DEMENTIA AND ALZHEIMER'S

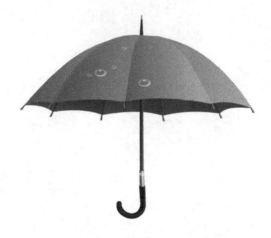

13

Personhood: The Heart of Your Well-being

Often, families and other care partners think they are doing the right thing for their loved ones by imposing burdensome treatments or interventions. But Dr. (Casarett) Karlawish suggests we ask family members what constitutes a good day even when a person has advanced dementia.

"We need to focus on what gives pleasure now, in the present," he says. This can be a challenge, but it's an important one. "When individuals have dementia, their lives—their very selves—are constructed by the people around them. We shape their personhood, and that is a tremendous moral responsibility."

—Chris Laxton, Executive Director of the AMDA

The concept of personhood is likely to be new to you because, until now, it hasn't been relevant. You know that you are a complete, conscious, functioning adult person. Your friends and family also know this. Your personhood is something that is taken for granted in Earth-reality.

Dementia complicates things, not because you are less of a person, but because as Alzheimer's progresses, it may become more difficult for your caregivers and others to relate to you. This is a common problem for anyone with a handicap, and especially for someone who appears to have reduced verbal or memory skills. It is all too easy for friends and family to regard an individual with Alzheimer's as being childlike or "diminished" in a manner that makes them less than a complete person. This is often not intentional but a consequence of not understanding how to relate to them, which, in part, is based on the stigma that society attaches to dementia.

In the early and middle stages of Alzheimer's, this can be very annoying; no one likes being treated like a child or a fool. In the later stages, it can be devastating, because the lack of connection with you as a person can negatively affect communication and caregiving. It's possible you may have already noticed this attitude coming from well-meaning family and friends who don't fully understand what you are experiencing. How do you overcome this bias?

The concept of *personhood* helps. It reminds everyone, including you, that dementia does not change the importance of respecting your integrity as an adult human being. *Maintaining your core sense of self as a compete person is vital for your well-being.* It is also the bottom line for your caregivers. You are and always will be, first, *you*, the person they know—and second, someone with dementia.

The Origin of Personhood

Personhood is a concept that was originally developed by psychologist Tom Kitwood in 1999, to remind professional staff and caregivers that *diminished everyday living skills do not make an individual less of a person.* Honoring personhood is respecting an individual's right to be perceived and treated as an adult in all situations. As a person with dementia, you obviously will want this kind of respect.

Being elderly and needing special assistance because of your age presents some role-related challenges that can be confusing to caregivers and others. Dementia only makes these role conflicts more complicated. These are gray areas because people, even professionals who know better, will confuse diminished verbal or memory skills with reduced mental functioning and, without intending harm, be demeaning or disrespectful. To prevent this from happening, I want to give you the tools to make sure that your caregivers understand the concept of personhood and the rules for how to preserve it.

Person-centered Care

To understand these rules, I need to introduce one more idea, that of *person-centered care*. Put simply, person-centered care is the operational side of personhood. Person-centered care describes how family and friends need to behave to offer maximum respect for your personhood. Many traditional, professional-driven approaches to dementia care focus on specific treatments, tasks, or procedures, rather than on you and the quality of your life. Alzheimer's research, treatment programs, guidebooks for family and staff, and institutional policies often follow this practice-driven paradigm. On the other hand, at its core, person-centered care is about honoring *you* as an individual who has something to say and needs to be met—essentially the same things we all might expect from any close friend.

What choice will you make? Probably it will be for person-centered care. You will want your caregivers and others to focus less on the mechanics of living with Alzheimer's and more on you—what you need, what you are experiencing, and what can be done to add positive moments to your life. To make this happen, you may need to give them some help. They will not suddenly wake up one morning and understand what to do! The good news is that many books and free materials that describe the details of person-centered care also include concrete suggestions to guide your caregivers.

One of the best guides I have seen comes from an excellent article by Timothy Epp, titled "Person-centered Dementia Care: A Vision to be Refined," published in the *Canadian Alzheimer Disease Review* in 2003. Here is an abbreviated version of his guidelines.

Recognition: Your caregivers greet you, say your name, make eye contact, and speak to you.

Negotiation: Your caregivers consult with you about choices and preferences.

Collaboration: Your caregivers work with you to complete tasks or projects.

Play: Your caregivers play games or engage in other activities that encourage you to have fun and be spontaneous.

Stimulation: Your caregivers help to engage you in activities that use all of your senses.

Celebration: Your caregivers find ways to celebrate something that you enjoy.

Relaxation: Your caregivers provide physical comfort and touch.

Validation: Your caregivers acknowledge your emotions and feelings with an empathetic response.

Holding: Your caregivers provide a comfortable space for you to open up without fear or concern about evaluation.

Facilitation: Your caregivers work with you to focus on what you can do, not areas where you are challenged.

Creation: Your caregivers encourage you to offer something spontaneously to your interactions.

Giving: Your caregivers encourage you to offer help or a positive attitude in your interactions.

This list contains the tools that your caregivers may need to support your sense of personhood throughout the Alzheimer's process. Please remind them that it is much more helpful for them to support "who you are now" than to spend a lot of time remembering "who you used to be." I recommend that you share these ideas with them, and also encourage them to connect with the Dementia Action Alliance online (daanow.org) for examples of how these tools are used by families and professionals.

KEY POINTS

- The concept of personhood is likely to be new to you because it is taken for granted in pre-dementia reality. You know and your friends and family know that you a complete, adult person.

- Dementia can change things, not because you are less of a person but because others may see you as diminished in some way or childlike.

- The concept of personhood reminds everyone, including you, that dementia does not change your identity as an independent, adult human being who expects to be supported by care partners but always treated as an adult.

- Personhood is a concept that was originally developed by psychologist Tom Kitwood in 1999 as an alternative to institutional, treatment-driven approaches to dementia care.

- Person-centered care is the operational side of personhood. It describes how staff, family, and friends need to behave to offer maximum respect for your personhood.

- Timothy Epp offers a excellent set of guidelines, listed in this chapter, to help you educate others about person-centered care.

Ideas for your life? How might you act on them? What is the first step?

14

Learning to Live in Long Moments

Most of our adult lives are ruled by habits...from that cup of coffee in the morning until the 10 o'clock news. To a large degree they are mindless mechanisms that push our rudders left and right and fill the day without requiring much awareness or attention.

Over time, the progression of Alzheimer's replaces these habits with repetitive patterns, also mindless but much less purposeful and responsive to what is happening in the world.

Habits and patterns define the routines of the day—look for routines that work for you, that make things go more smoothly.

—Richard Fenker

The Long Moment: Communicating with the Alzheimer's Mind

The concept of a "long moment" comes from the self-reported experiences of many individuals living with dementia and from my earlier book on communication and Alzheimer's. In pre-dementia Earth-reality, time is an unbroken continuum that weaves itself into all of our experiences in a typical day. From morning until night, we have a clear sense of where we are along this continuum and how all of the events of the day are connected with it. There is no doubt that when you walk to the train in the morning, you are heading for work or shopping—or that on your return trip, you are headed home. Walking into the grocery store is linked with the dinner you are planning later, and the wine purchase makes it a special occasion. The bathrobe you wear before bedtime is found on the door, exactly where you left it hanging in the morning. The conversation with your spouse about a coming wedding picks up over dinner where you ended it before leaving for work. Time and the events of the day are part of a seamless panorama that in its familiarity goes largely unobserved and taken for granted.

Living with dementia changes everything! Brian LeBlanc, with early-onset Alzheimer's, is known for his polished, professional talks. However, his wife Shannon describes what these presentations don't reveal:

- *They, your audience, don't see who you are when you are away from the spotlight.*

- *They don't see the confusion, the anger, the anxiousness.*

- *They don't see the man who can't remember how to do the simplest of chores.*

- *They don't see the man who has a reminder on his phone to eat and to take a bath.*

- *They don't see the man who can't remember something he was told 5 or 10 minutes ago.*

- *They don't see the man who, without a prepared speech or notes, can't speak without stuttering or going blank.*

Dementia can change your experience of a series of connected events in time into a hodgepodge of disconnected chunks. You are thirsty and head to the kitchen for a glass of water— but a minute later, you are standing by the sink, wondering why you are there. This is the norm. On the other hand, when events are well-structured with proper reminders or memory bridges, the chunks can be much longer. I recently spent an hour with Brian on a conference call with no sense of gaps or any other clues that would suggest a problem with memory or concentration.

Defining a Long Moment

A "long moment" is simply a unit of time in the world of dementia that defines a single, focused activity or event. It may last only a few seconds, a few minutes or an hour—that depends on the person and the nature of the activity. My video call with Brian, for example, was filled with clues to keep him engaged and remind him of the context. Once that moment has finished, however, it is likely to be lost and not remembered as the individual moves on to the next activity or "moment." Earth-reality is also full of long moments, but typically they are all connected in the sequence that we define as a day. Life for someone with dementia is essentially a sequence of *disconnected* long moments or blocks of time.

It is important to realize that while your experience of time is likely to change with Alzheimer's, as short-term memory loss brings more and more of your experience into the present tense, the units of time that really matter, long moments, will be essentially the same as in your previous life. Connected in a sequence or not, most of our living is done in these chunks of time. When we think of the *concept* of time, we may be thinking of units such as days or weeks or years, but our *experience* of time tends to take place now, in the moment. Because of this, our judgments about the quality of our experiences in time are often judgments about long moments. This was true in your pre-dementia past, it is true now, and it will be even truer later in the Alzheimer's journey, when the tendency of your mind to ruminate about the past or fret about the future vanishes.

Living in the present means literally "living in the moment" with the units of living that define what you experience in your conscious mind being essentially long moments. There is really nothing else. You can describe a sequence of long moments, for example, as a longer unit of time such as "a day." But this is an abstraction. Good days and bad days are really about the quality of the long moments that you experience during this period.

An Exercise in "Ideal Time"

Let me give you an example from my own life to clarify this concept. In my college class, States of Consciousness, I used an exercise called "Ideal Time" with the students. Their assignment the first week was to plan and then experience whatever they would define as an "Ideal Minute" and then write a one-paragraph report on this episode. No one experienced any difficulty with this first task and, as you might expect, I received an array of reports about many pleasurable activities, including long kisses, smoking a joint, and eating ice cream.

In the second week, the task was to plan and experience an "Ideal Hour." Once again, this presented little problem and most students loved the idea of planning and doing something that was enjoyable as part of an assignment.

You may have already guessed the third week's exercise, which was to plan and experience an "Ideal Day." It was at this point that the process began to break down for many students. Reports this week often communicated the frustration of wanting to do the assignment but quickly recognizing that it was not realistic, at least with their current interpretation of "ideal," to spend a whole day out of a busy week on this project.

By the time I gave the final assignment, to plan and experience an "Ideal Week" and report on the results, the real point of the exercise was obvious to most students. If ideal time is based solely on pleasure and enjoyment, then the opportunities for living an ideal day are challenging, and to live an ideal week, impossible! Now, with this background, I was able to introduce the notion that ideal time is really about *how you experience all moments in time, pleasurable or not.* It is your response to these moments, not how much you enjoy them in a literal sense, that matters.

If you go through life defining ideal time strictly in terms of pleasure and enjoyment, there is likely to be lots of down time that isn't ideal. On the other hand, if you define time in a manner that is anchored to the moment and to your responses to that moment, virtually all time can be "ideal" and experienced as happy, enjoyable, and fulfilling.

How We Remember the Past

Our perception of the past, especially our history, tends to be an illusion. Much research suggests that we don't remember a continuum of time filled with a sequence of events. Instead, what we typically recall are key moments that highlight our highs and lows—with the remainder of our history falling into the "meantime" category. We remember, for example, the result of a close game when our home team won or lost, and we may also recall the key play that made a difference. We remember the moment we became engaged. We remember the loss of a close friend or family member and the pain we experienced. In brief, we remember the peaks and valleys of our lives, often with a fortunate bias toward those moments that were positive in nature.

Looking forward from the perspective of your life *before* Alzheimer's, you can choose to see your future as days or weeks or years of "non-ideal" time, which is one common view. You can also change this perspective to create a different future, one that isn't biased by the past but based instead on what you actually will experience. By breaking life down into a sequence of long moments, you will find that the substance of living a full life completely and joyfully can be found in these moments.

Richard Taylor describes his own focus here:

I appreciate and sometimes immerse myself in the process rather than only or mostly on the outcome. I like doing things. I like and appreciate the doing. Doing is how I know I am alive. I appreciate being alive.

Although you and your caregivers may not be able to affect the physical changes that take place with Alzheimer's, you can change the quality of many of the moments you experience. This is not a wish but an objective fact, demonstrated continuously by the work of thousands of professional and family caregivers. The catch is that, to make many of these coming moments meaningful and joyful, you will have to "let go" of expectations in Earth-reality that push you to be verbal, logical, and not make mistakes—and instead, relax and accept what comes next. Most likely this will happen naturally without your doing anything. You just won't care as much about what is happening around you because it doesn't matter. This is good and represents a landmark on your journey.

When you and your caregivers agree that one of your goals is to add thousands of meaningful, positive moments to your life, it will happen. By focusing on the moment, not on a day or a vague future, you bring the process for managing the experiences in your life into a practical context. During a difficult period, can I, as a care partner, change a tough day into a good one? Probably not. Can I do concrete things like listening, soothing frustration, entertaining, helping you laugh—all of which add quality long moments? Yes, I can. What are these concrete things accomplishing? They are transforming bad moments into good ones.

Habits and Patterns

In your life before Alzheimer's, typically it is *habits* that dominate the majority of your long moments—and the lives of most other adults. From that cup of coffee in the morning until you hit the bed at night, most of your behavior consists of habit-driven routines that require very little conscious activity or monitoring. This leaves the full power of your conscious mind for the few things that *do* demand your attention, like a grizzly bear in your kitchen. To a large degree, these habits are learned, mindless mechanisms that guide you through the day with a minimum of cognitive activity.

Habits that you sustain throughout your journey with dementia make great allies, because they provide the structure for many positive, familiar, routine moments. Drinking coffee in the morning, watching the weather on TV, dining, walking in the garden—and the sequence of other activities that take you through the day—place precious boundaries around your time that can help you orient. A habit offers a launching ramp to a period of non-thinking good time when the symptoms of dementia are kept at bay. Habits are probably the largest source of quality long moments in your life, before and after dementia, so look to maintain them in the future.

Habits are your friends because they take place in normal time. Dressing, drinking coffee, and watching the news are behaviors connected with the dimension of time, because they are constrained by physical reality. You cannot say "poof" and magically be dressed, or instantly teleport from the bedroom to the living room. These activities have to unfold over time to be successful.

Patterns, on the other hand, are a form of unconscious habit that can appear as your dementia progresses. They are much less friendly, not so much to you (because you will not notice them) as to your caregivers. Patterns are repetitive behaviors that signal a breakdown in your short-term memory. Essentially, you may not remember that the behavior you are starting now has been repeated several times before. Pattern-based habits signal a disconnect between the sequence of behaviors and the time dimension in Earth-reality. Time is no longer a continuum for you but is divided into a set of discrete chunks, separate from each other. Each new moment wakes you up as if the previous moments did not exist.

Image a record with your favorite music (yes, I know you are old enough to remember vinyl records). While most of the record and the beautiful music it contains in the grooves remains intact, over time, scratches appear. Each time the needle hits a scratch, it jumps up, bounces back to a previous set of grooves and starts again. This is your mind when it is caught in a repetitive cycle of pattern behavior.

Reducing Pattern Behavior

This doesn't sound like fun, even if you aren't aware of it. What can you do about it? I recommend five things:

1. Use established habits to sustain your connection with Earth-time.

2. Engage in behaviors that activate the parts of your mind that can support connections over time. Singing or listening to music or playing certain games or even walking can keep the time dimension unbroken for long periods.

3. Use a wake-up routine to help you orient when there is a break in time.

4. Use habit reminders and other tools to remind you that the activity you are doing has a sequence of steps—and to help you identify where you are in the sequence.

5. Remember the record example above? What would you do if you were playing this record? You would simply pick up the needle and move it past the scratches to another part of the record. Ask your caregivers to do the same. When pattern behavior begins, instead of ignoring it, they can move you to another part of the record by changing topics or changing places or beginning a well-established habit. Even with the scratches, most of you is still somewhere on that record.

Doses of reality are precious breaks in a day filled with too many habits-becoming-patterns. They add joy and positive moments and can help block recycling patterns. Visits to a garden, a store, a museum, a restaurant, or a sporting event offer stimulation and familiarity plus rules and boundaries that are not dementia-related.

Overcoming feelings of helplessness and frustration with dementia is all about intentionality. When you can effectively exercise your willpower to get what you want and need, even in the smallest of ways, you are strengthening your intentionality muscle—the key to having a measure of choice and independence in your life. The next chapter offers a simple but powerful tool to help.

KEY POINTS

- Normal time in Earth-reality is a seamless, connected series of blocks of time linked to the past, present, and future but always experienced in the present.

- Dementia-time also consists of a series of blocks or chunks of time but because of short-term memory loss, they are often *disconnected*.

- A "long moment" is a brief unit of time that defines a single focused activity or event. It may last a few seconds, a few minutes, or even an hour, in some cases. Both normal and dementia-time are filled with long moments.

- Because dementia brings more and more of your experience into the present tense, life with dementia becomes a sequence of disconnected long moments lived in the present.

- When you find ways to interpret these long moments as positive or at least neutral (versus interpreting them negatively), you add a great deal of quality or "ideal time" to your life.

- Everyday habits often dominate our lives from that first cup of coffee in the morning to brushing your teeth before bed at night. Habits are great allies on the Alzheimer's journey because they are typically positive or neutral and can bridge long moments into a sequence.

- Pattern behavior, which is common with dementia, represents unconscious, repetitive habits. This is less of a problem for you than your caregivers, who may need some education to support you properly.

Ideas for your life? How might you act on them? What is the first step?

15

Adding Joy and Intentionality with a Bucket List

I turned the big 60 this year. I need to go back and review my bucket list. My son gave me one of the items on my bucket list: "an IOU for a skydiving trip." Something I have always wanted to do—we were going to try it last year but the timing didn't work out for us. He has promised this will be the year.

I am grateful to be doing as well as I am. Still trying to stay active, and keep the brain active as well. I have really had to say "no" a lot this year to give myself some breathing room. Activities wear me out quickly so I have to cut back on some things—but I am still plugging along.

—Kris, from her blog, *Dealing with Alzheimer's*

To a generation of movie fans, *The Bucket List* is a movie starring Jack Nicholson and Morgan Freeman. The idea of creating a list of things you would like to do before you "kick the bucket" has been around for many years, however, as part of workshops and self-help programs.

It's not a bad idea. Why? Because creating a bucket list makes a powerful statement to the universe that you plan to keep on living. In fact, you plan to live long enough to do all of the things on the list!

A typical bucket list might read something like the illustration on the next page.

My Bucket List

1. Experience the Northern Lights
2. See an osprey in the wild
3. Walk the Worcestershire Way trail
4. Write my memoirs
5. Go whale watching
6. Learn to play the piano
7. Ride a gondola in Venice
8. Take the children to a football match
9. Tell grandad I love him

Now, let's think for a moment about *your* bucket list. I can hear your mind churning. Wait a minute, you are thinking, I am way too old to have a bucket list and besides, I have Alzheimer's.

Good try, but I'm not about to let you off the hook that easy. Of course you have Alzheimer's. That's why you are reading this book instead of *Sports Illustrated* or *Vogue*. It's also why you need a bucket list, right now.

You have decided to live life fully despite having dementia. Creating your bucket list is a big first step in that direction. Do you think you're too old for a bucket list? Think again. Your age and living situation don't matter. There are always things within your reach, things that you can plan to do with the help of family and friends.

Here is a somewhat less-ambitious list, in case you are not ready to do more globetrotting.

- Thank my family
- Visit all of the museums in my city
- Go sailing on a local lake
- Surprise my spouse with a gift every day for a week
- Have doughnuts for breakfast

Does this seem to fit your lifestyle better?

My Aunt Emilou was 90 when she was diagnosed with Alzheimer's. Can you guess what she wanted to do? Two things. She wanted a vacation where the extended family all got together again so she could see everyone while she remembered them. Wish granted. We rented three houses on the bay at Fripp Island and had a wonderful week. Second wish: She had been hearing of cruises for many years but had never been on one. Her daughter Katherine took her for a week to the Caribbean, which she loved.

I want your list to be longer than the samples above, with at least 15 to 20 items. They don't need to be big things or things that don't make sense given your budget. My mom at 88 wanted to go to a concert performed by the Fort Worth Symphony. She also wanted to see the wonderful Botanical Gardens. Both were things Dad did not want to do, so she used this as an opportunity to go with a group of friends from the retirement center. These may not seem like much, but both trips for her were adventures! They fit her lifestyle and brought a big smile to her face.

What fits your lifestyle and interests? My mom's visits were easy options but also perfect for a bucket list because they represented things she would never do without a push. Since you know that Alzheimer's will affect your short-term memory at some point in the future, are there things you would like to do with family and friends now? Are there places you want to visit? Museums are a great resource for people with dementia, at all stages. What about family you would like to see? It may be a good idea to get your caregivers involved as you make your list since, for many items, they will be supporting you.

Your bucket list and your happiness checklist (the things that make you happy every day) are closely related. It's fine to move items from one list to another. What starts as a big goal (such as watching a TV series on the Civil War) can become an everyday goal when divided into many parts.

Making your bucket list is a big and important first step in acknowledging your choice to live a complete and joyful life. Every item is a reminder that you are celebrating many of the moments in your life, not watching passively as they drift by. Have fun!

KEY POINTS

- Living a full life with dementia means in part living a life that finds happiness and joy in the things that you do each day.

- A bucket list is simply a list of things that you would like to do before you die.

- Creating a bucket list makes a powerful statement to the universe that you intend to keep on living.

- Being older and having Alzheimer's will not stop you from creating a bucket list. You may be visiting a museum or dining at Four Seasons instead of climbing Mount Everest, but that's OK.

- Create a bucket list that fits your lifestyle and get to work checking off the items. Challenge your care partners to see that you do everything on the list!

- Your bucket list and happiness checklist (from Chapter 2) are closely related.

- Making your bucket list is a big and important first step in acknowledging your choice to live a complete and joyful life. Every item is a reminder that you are celebrating many of the moments in your life, not watching passively as they drift by.

Ideas for your life? How might you act on them? What is the first step?

16

Using Affirmations to Tune Your Consciousness

Be kind, always.
Spend time on your passion; if you don't know what it is, work on finding it.
Tell the important people in your life how much you love them.
Take more walks.
Spend time with friends; reconnect with someone you haven't seen
  in a long time.
Worry less.
Believe in yourself and your worth.
Embrace creative pursuits.

    —Ann Napoletan, from her blog *The Long and Winding Road*

The last several chapters have focused on specific things you can do to live a full life: Embrace your personhood, live in long moments, and create a bucket list. This chapter brings all these ideas together and supercharges them with the power of affirmation.

Affirmations are short reminders that you give yourself to orient your self-talk in the best possible directions. Self-talk? Yes, it's a fact. You constantly talk to yourself about what you are thinking, feeling, and experiencing. Wait a minute. If you're talking, who's listening? You are. There is a talking part of your mind and another part that listens. Because no one filters these conversations, you tend to believe what you say to yourself! Now that is a scary thought, because it means that your self-talk, to a large degree, becomes your reality.

Think for a moment about the conversations taking place in your mind since the Alzheimer's diagnosis. Are they positive and focused on overcoming the challenges that the disease presents, or are they negative and pessimistic? It's impossible to be 100 percent positive while you are still grieving, but having some portion of your thoughts be positive is very important. Why? Because your world is not a fixed, immutable thing but something you create at every moment in your mind. Positive thoughts expressed as words you say to yourself have tremendous power to shape your experience with dementia.

Affirmations for Dementia

Here are some helpful affirmations for living a complete and joyful life with Alzheimer's or another type of dementia:

- I accept completely the fact that I have dementia. I do not judge this positively or negatively. It is just my reality.

- I gently let go of any negative reaction my family or I might have to this diagnosis. I move on positively and engage with my life.

- I focus on the quality of the long moments I am experiencing. In this way, I live a complete and joyful life throughout the Alzheimer's process.

- I strive to keep my mind and body active and engaged in living every day.

- I relinquish the need to follow the social conventions and rules of Earth-reality.

- I am a complete, independent, adult person now and will continue to be so for the rest of my life. I expect others to honor and support the integrity of my personhood, which is so vital to me.

- I love and trust my caregivers. I strive to accept and benefit from their caring, even though at times I may not understand them or their intentions.

- I choose to have as much independence as possible at all stages of the Alzheimer's process.

- I embrace technology and other tools that enhance the quality of my life.

- I make important health, financial, legal, and social decisions as early as possible, to unburden myself and others.

- I embrace my life with gratitude. I am blessed to be alive, aware, and supported by so many kind people.

Please realize that this collection of affirmations is not a complete list or necessarily the best list for you. You probably will have others you want to add that fit your needs and lifestyle. What are the thoughts and statements you can make that will help to focus your mind on positive outcomes?

When you finish your list, what do you do with these affirmations? You make them a part of your consciousness by reading them to yourself daily or by having someone read them to you. They support your happiness and well-being without your even being aware this is happening. Affirmations tune your conscious and unconscious mind to find and experience the reality they represent. What you say to yourself to a large degree *creates* the reality you experience, with or without a diagnosis of Alzheimer's. When you flip through the radio stations looking for news or country music or pop songs, that is what you find. When you tune your mind to look for joyful moments and a positive approach to Alzheimer's, that is also what you will find.

Often your self-talk is associated with the thinking part of your mind. Your feelings about the world follow your thoughts. If your thoughts are happy (or sad, angry, grateful, frustrated, and so forth), your feelings will have the same flavor. Tuning your mind, by using the words you say to yourself to direct your emotions, is powerful and effective.

You have already made the choice (in Chapter 1) to live life to its fullest. The affirmations listed above are some of the most powerful tools available to make this happen. You may already be experiencing some noise and confusion in your mind as you think about your current situation. Your affirmations help by cutting through this noise to keep you tuned to the right stations. Accepting that you have Alzheimer's can help you move through much of the grief you and your family may be feeling at this moment. Giving yourself permission not to follow the rules that are part of the old world allows you to regard your lapses more lightly and without judgment.

The steps you are taking to continue to live your life as a parade will serve you well. But there is more to do, now, while your mind is still healthy. What you say to yourself has a strong impact on what you will experience but so do your emotions, especially the feelings of frustration and anger that often accompany dementia. How do you deal with these feelings? The next chapter covers this important topic.

KEY POINTS

- Self-talk is the running conversation you have in your mind with yourself about what you are thinking, feeling, and experiencing.

- Affirmations are short reminders that you give yourself to orient your self-talk in the best possible directions.

- To a large degree, your self-talk creates the world you experience. If it is optimistic and positive, the world is a friendly place. If it is negative, you may be struggling in an unfriendly world.

- You can make your world, living with dementia, a more positive place by making your self-talk more positive. Affirmations are an excellent way to do this.

- Here is one example of a simple affirmation that you might read to yourself on a regular basis: *I choose to have as much independence as possible at all stages of the Alzheimer's process.*

- The affirmation "tunes" your self-talk so that unconsciously, it becomes a part of how you view the world. You want independence? *You are independent.*

- You have already made the choice to live life to its fullest. Your affirmations help make this possible by cutting through the noise to keep you tuned to the right stations.

Ideas for your life? How might you act on them? What is the first step?

17

Embracing Your Anger

One of the things that makes me angry about having Alzheimer's Disease are people that DO NOT WANT TO UNDERSTAND that I, and people like me, still know what's going on around them and can still carry on an intelligent conversation. Sure, the words may not flow as evenly and smoothly as they did before, the mind may not allow us to remember the conversation an hour or a day or a week from now, but we still enjoy being in the moment.
—Brian LeBlanc, from his blog *Alzheimer's: The Journey*

I'm sure I don't need to tell you about anger. No one can move through the stages of Alzheimer's or any other form of dementia without feeling a healthy dose of anger and frustration. Anger and dementia go hand in hand. The community of professionals and caregivers familiar with the problem acknowledges that it is a major issue; however, their focus is really not on you and the cause of the anger but on what they need to do to manage the situation. There are books full of suggestions for how to calm you or prevent such outbursts. Meanwhile, what you needed to say may not be heard or understood.

This chapter isn't for the community that supports you. It's for you. Let me begin by saying that your anger is a normal and healthy expression of what is happening inside your mind.

It may not be convenient for your caregivers and others, who would love for you to be passive and happy and cooperative, but that is not to be. From your perspective, the anger is a natural outlet for the frustrations you are bound to feel in living with dementia. In other words, it's good. Think of it as the energy needed to drive the messages that you want to send to the world.

The real purpose for managing your anger is not to provide benefits for your caregivers but benefits for you. Anger and frustration may be inconvenient, but they aren't bad. They are your fuel for releasing and communicating some of what you are feeling on the dementia journey. The key is to find the balance that allows anger to work for you and for your caregivers.

"Wait a minute," you may be thinking. "If I'm angry, I have the right to release that anger and frustration in any way I want. In fact, I may not be able to control it. After all, I do have dementia." Good try. Yes, you have dementia, but you are a complete, intelligent, independent person living with dementia, not a robot. You have a lot of control over your anger and how to use it to add positive, long moments to your life.

How do you accomplish this? I have five suggestions for you.

Embrace Your Anger

You've earned the right to be angry or frustrated! Like millions who suffer from ailments that impede communication, such as stroke, you live in a world where what you know and want to say is too often trapped inside you. The thought or need is clear in your mind but cannot cross the left-brain speech barrier to become a coherent, logical statement that your caregivers will understand. In some cases, the *right* words in your mind become the *wrong* words when spoken. The pace of the conversation may race past your internal clock, so that before you can respond others have completed the sentence or compromised your independence by taking the action you wanted to take.

You have the right to be angry! Now what do you do want to do about it? To begin with, *nothing*. You can feel the anger and frustration. That's good. It means you're still alive and well. You may want to do something to release it in a moment, but to begin with, you just notice it. You can say to yourself, "I'm angry," or any other words that express what you're feeling. Remember, you're in control here. This is your world. You notice the anger and for a moment, just embrace it and recognize that you have this feeling. You can do this. Sometimes it helps to associate the feeling with a color, such as red; a sound, such as a bell that rings in your mind; or a physical action, such as clenching your fist. All of these cues can help anchor the experience of being angry and delay your response for a few seconds.

Signal to Your Caregivers

Imagine for a moment that, every time you begin to feel angry about something when you are with your caregivers, you find a way to signal this anger to them (other than exploding). There are many good nonverbal signals; try raising your hand, closing your eyes, putting on a special hat, or using a stuffed animal. Two important things happen when you do this. First, the signal prepares your mind to communicate a message, even if that message is just the fact that you are angry. Second, it tells your caregivers that you have something to say and that you want them to tune into your wavelength.

In some current treatment approaches, such a signal would mean, "Look out, George is about to explode. Let's prepare by going into anger management mode." In my approach, which represents you and not your caregivers, the signal means that you have something to say and that your anger is a positive thing, the energy behind the communication.

Make the Communication

Let it rip! Say or do, using words, cards, objects, or hand signals, what you want to communicate, no matter how ugly the process. You want a glass of water but you keep saying "Waltz." You want extra time to decide what to order from the take-out menu but pointing to the menu confuses your caregivers. You are really annoyed that your spouse left this morning to go to church without you but can only express this with anger, not words. Sometimes you can communicate your needs, but many times you can't. That's OK. You have done your part and now your listeners need to do some work to interpret your messages.

Look for a Response that Says You Were Understood

We all appreciate, at any time in our lives, someone who really listens to us. It's even more satisfying if that someone also shows us, through an "active listening" process, that what we said was heard and understood. Typically, this means repeating back to us what the listener heard us say. It is a very powerful communication tool. In the context of dementia, active listening covers a much broader area than verbal communication. It may include meeting a need you expressed, acknowledging your feelings, or just getting in tune with where you happen to be at the moment.

When you are not understood, you can use the energy from your anger to persist. Keep your hand raised (if this is your signal) to indicate that the process is not finished. You still have something to say. In books and blog posts by individuals with dementia, a common theme is the need to have others really listen in an active manner, by focusing less on the words and more on deciphering the meaning of what the person is communicating.

Let Go of the Anger Once You are Heard

In some contexts today, it is assumed that the caregiver has successfully managed your anger when they have made a response that causes it to be reduced or to go away. That may not be your world. You may be ready to release the anger only when you are heard. The anger says you have something to say. Letting go of the anger acknowledges that your caregivers or others have listened and gotten the message, at least in part. If your signal for the communication was the raised hand, now you can lower it.

Appreciate the Challenge and Move on

Remember that your anger or frustration is often a good thing. It's the fuel that drives you to communicate to others that you need something. It is the antidote to passivity and helplessness. Anger is one of the most powerful tools available to you for reaching out to express your independence. Help your caregivers understand that, rather than avoiding or attempting to suppress this anger, they need to embrace it, listen to it, find ways to see the humor in it, and then use it as a basis for communication.

Many of the most important things in life are connected to the emotions we feel. Anger is just another emotion, but a very important one when it indicates that something you need to say or do is being blocked. Help your caregivers learn to manage your anger by focusing their attention on what is blocked and drawing it out, rather than by trying to suppress it.

You will feel anger and frustration many times on your journey. Learn to use it as an ally.

KEY POINTS

- Feeling angry or frustrated at times is a normal and healthy part of your experience with dementia.

- Most materials on anger, however, focus not on you but on what your caregivers need to do to *manage the situation* when you are upset. The real purpose for managing your anger is to provide benefits for you.

- Anger can provide the source of energy needed for you to release some of the bottled-up emotions that are part of your Alzheimer's journey.

- For anger to add quality to your life, not just more frustration, you need to find the balance between simply releasing it versus controlling it enough to enhance communications with your caregivers.

- Here is a five-step process for making anger and frustration work for you:

  1. **Embrace your anger:** Before you respond, simply recognize that you are angry and hold onto this feeling for a moment.

  2. **Signal it to your caregivers:** Work out a process for signaling anger to your caregivers. Raise your hand or close your eyes or make a fist. Find a signal that works for you.

  3. **Make a communication:** Use words or cards or sign language or any other form of communication to tell your caregivers what you want to say.

  4. **Look to see that you were understood:** Look for a sign that your message was heard by them.

  5. **Let go of the anger:** Now you can let go. Your message was communicated!

Ideas for your life? How might you act on them? What is the first step?

18

Helping Others Communicate

The fact is, most experts spend more time talking to and listening to caregivers than they do talking to and listening to those of us with dementia.
—Greg O'Brien, *On Pluto: Inside the Mind of Alzheimer's*

Perhaps the biggest challenge you will face during the Alzheimer's journey is communication. Many times, you will have something to say and others will not understand—and this can be very frustrating. Part of the problem is that your verbal skills will be affected; you may find it more difficult to put your thoughts into words and speak them. You will know or want things that are clear in your mind but difficult for you to communicate.

The other part of the problem is that in Earth-reality, we take communication with others for granted because we share the same world. Without even thinking about it, we "consensually validate" each other's experiences. Because we both know how to identify the color red on a stoplight, or judge that a cup of coffee will be hot, or to avoid dark alleys at night, we don't need to talk about these things. They are part of a complex, shared reality. With Alzheimer's, your reality will be different and in many cases *not* shared, so having a common framework for communication can't be taken for granted.

Richard Taylor shares his thoughts on this subject:

Perhaps too much time is spent trying to answer and question each other, when what I really need is to feel like I am being heard.

I am increasingly sensitive about myself. If people dare ask me a question, or appear not to understand me, I become defensive: "What do you mean you don't know what I mean? How many times do I have to tell you?"

The biggest challenge is not *your* problems in communicating, it's your caregivers'! They live in a world of words and memories and logic that they take for granted. You are going to need to give them a push and many reminders to help them join your reality. Learning to come to you and fully appreciate the boundaries of your world will take time and practice. It is much like learning a foreign language, except more difficult—because now, the same English words and expressions may have different meanings. Richard Taylor expresses his frustration here:

I speak to my caregivers and they seem to understand every word, every thought. Yet they do not behave as if they have heard me.

Listening to you speak *in your own language* is the most important skill for your caregivers to develop. They need to understand that it is not what you are saying that matters but how you are thinking about things. If you call a visitor George who is actually your friend Bob, it is probably not that you have confused the two but that Bob has elicited a feeling or memory associated with Uncle George. The message is about those feelings, not the people involved.

More than anything else, the goal of communication is for you to be heard. It takes time for your caregivers to learn how to do this, but with patience and this clear objective in mind they can be stars. A second important goal is to stay focused in the present time. Because caregivers often live in your past (they remember the pre-dementia you and have many associated memories), they may want to connect this past with you in the present. Remind them that it is much more helpful to support the *you* that is present right now than to pretend to be addressing the you from the past.

Having a real conversation about your experiences in living with Alzheimer's can be very challenging. This is difficult territory for family, physicians, and caregivers to explore. The frightening nature of the word "Alzheimer's" or "dementia" often blocks communication. A common response when I describe my work with dementia and the products I have created is an uncomfortable nod and the quickest escape possible. For caregivers to communicate effectively with you, they must cross the threshold into your territory. They must embrace your reality of living with dementia openly and frankly.

To accomplish this goal, it is vital for your caregivers to help remove any concern you might have about making mistakes. The fact is that you are going to be confused at times. You may start tasks and not remember why you started them. You may misplace things that are right in front of you. You may be reduced at times to guessing the names of objects or people. All of this is normal; it comes with the territory as dementia interferes with your thinking and behavior. However, it is easy for others to make it a problem through their tendency to evaluate, criticize, or act impatient. These responses only feed your anxieties about "doing things wrong."

In fact, it won't take much of this type of feedback to destroy communication by making you fearful of speaking out. Remind your caregivers to listen for what you intend to communicate, *not the words you are speaking.* Ask them to encourage and support you, not offer corrections and criticism. With some practice, I'm sure they will be up to the task.

Here are some approaches you and your caregivers might use to help you communicate.

Find Alternatives to Speaking

Realize that you have many resources other than speech to communicate. Writing, pointing, using a chart with images, making gestures, touching, or employing a simple sign language can all be good alternatives. It can be frustrating to want to speak and discover that the right words won't come. Learn to relax, forgive your disability, and find another way to make your communication happen.

Educate Your Caregivers

Our culture is so dependent on speech that one of your biggest challenges will be to help your caregivers understand that they need to learn to use alternate modalities, too. They will need to learn to come to you, rather than expecting you to come to them. What this means in practical terms is they need to stop trying to pull you back into their reality—Earth-reality—by demanding that you think and communicate logically, sequentially and verbally. Pressuring you to "say what you are thinking" or to remember your past is simply not fair. It reflects a kind of laziness or inattention on their part. A little education should quickly fix this problem.

Focus on the Moment

It is easy to lose the thread of a conversation when the context changes. In Earth-reality, we jump from topic to topic and context to context without thinking about it. Focus on one thing and communicate that one idea before moving on; then listen to be certain the message was heard.

Use the Communication Cards and Apps

The Alzheimer's Communication Cards and other tools that are part of products such as Amazon's Echo or the personal assistants available on smartphones work well for general communications and can be customized to create messages that are specific to your circumstances. The Communication Cards, for example, allow you to think about a message you need to communicate, find the appropriate card, and share it with others. This is a tool you will be able to use throughout the dementia process.

Slow Down

It can be hard not to become frustrated and impatient when you have tried to communicate something important and your caregivers have not understood. Slow down. The real problem is likely to be your caregivers not listening because they have slipped back into Earth-reality and forgotten to come to you. Help them understand by relaxing and finding the best alternative to speech to communicate your message.

Several person-centered organizations have created guidelines for helping your family and caregivers communicate more effectively with you. You will find some of these listed in the online resources I've included in Appendix B.

Silence as the Default Setting

Silence is a big part of Alzheimer's. Of the 18.1 billion caregiver hours donated last year, probably more than half were spent in silence. *You* may want to be silent, if the context has an edge of evaluation to it, so that you avoid making mistakes. "Memory testing" or any other kind of competency testing tends to create this type of environment. *Your caregivers* may want to be quiet because of their own issues with competence. They may not know what to do or say in many situations. Given this uncertainty, if being silent promotes an atmosphere where you appear to be content, so much the better, as far as they are concerned. The worst case for them is to say something that will provoke or upset you. That experience could quickly shut down future conversations, so often silence rules—even when contact and emotion are just what you need most.

How do you deal with this problem? A good start might be to share with your caregivers the recommendations for improving communication described above. The communication guidelines in the table below also contain many helpful ideas to support better interactions with caregivers. Having these guidelines available means that your caregivers are no longer at a loss and forced to resort to silence by default. Fixing their insecurity is just as important as addressing your own. The challenge for you is to learn and learn and learn again to let go of the conflict you feel inside when you do or say something that is not correct, complete, or appropriate. That may be part of who you are now, living with dementia, and it is OK. Turning loose these words and behaviors is much healthier than smothering them in silence and discomfort.

Solving communication problems is essential to living a complete and joyful life. Your independence and the quality of the many long moments you experience will depend on this. One key to communicating is to let go of the need to do everything with words and use other options. The next chapter expands on this idea by recommending that you let go of many other requirements of Earth-reality.

Care Partner Communication Guidelines

Dear Family and Friends, I'm going to need your help to continue to communicate effectively. Please use the following guidelines.

• Find a quiet place. Turn off the TV. Distractions you take for granted are very challenging for me.

• Please be patient with me. It may take some time for me to communicate what I need to say or to understand you.

• Focus on my feelings first, then on the logic of what I am trying to communicate. Both are important, but if I'm feeling unhappy or frustrated for any reason, then this takes priority.

• Please don't argue with me or try to correct me. Be supportive and listen. Ask questions to learn more.

• Address me directly by looking at me and speaking my name to let me know you have something to communicate.

- Speak slowly and distinctly with a clear message in mind. I probably will not understand vague or complex statements. Please remember, though, that I am an adult, not a child.

- Negatives like "don't" are difficult for me to understand. Please try to express what I need to do, not what to avoid.

- Please don't quiz or test me. It is OK to share a memory, but never put me under pressure to recall or relate to it.

- At times, showing me a picture or words on paper will work much better than speaking to me.

KEY POINTS

- Communication with others is likely to be the biggest challenge on your journey with dementia. You will know what you need to say but may not be able to make others understand.

- Alzheimer's complicates things because you no longer share the same world with your family and friends. Your world depends less on words and logic and more on feelings.

- Your friends will need to come to you to make the communication process work, not attempt to pull you back to their world.

- Making mistakes is a normal, healthy part of communication when you have dementia. It is important to let go of your concerns about these errors, accept them, and not judge yourself.

- Keeping a sense of humor here is very helpful.

- Some simple things that your friends and family can do to enhance communication include:

  Go beyond speaking. Use pictures or gestures or touch.

  Learn how to communicate using the guidelines in this chapter.

  Focus on one thing at a time. Stay in the moment.

  Use available tools such as Communication Cards or applications designed to help.

  Go slow. Be patient.

  Embrace silence. It is a good and healthy part of the communication process.

Ideas for your life? How might you act on them? What is the first step?

19

Letting Go of Earth-reality

I live in my own little world, but it's OK ... they know me here.
—John Sandblom
EarlyOnsetAtypicalAlzheimersDisease.com/blog

L iving with Alzheimer's or any form of dementia can be very challenging in many social situations. The combination of expectations and judgment creates a great deal of pressure. You are expected to know how to behave when you meet friends, go to church, talk with colleagues about a project, or have dinner in a restaurant. Because strong social norms guide behavior in these situations, your own behavior is subject to evaluation. Alzheimer's is also challenging personally as you put pressure on yourself to think and function in pre-dementia ways and then cannot. These are all examples of conscious, ego-driven behaviors. The conflict you're experiencing here is based on the difference between your behavior in the world and your expectations or comparisons with pre-dementia behavior.

This chapter looks at the concept of letting go the natural tendency to try and live up to the expectations of others and ourselves—if you choose—and enjoying the benefits that come from simply being yourself.

Pushing and Letting Go

Most of us, living in Earth-reality, spend a great deal of our lives striving for success or at least demonstrating our capability to function well in this world. We want to be accepted by our friends and family, and appreciated for our contributions at work, and to have the feeling of self-confidence that comes when we are able to influence this reality in ways that work for us. Intentionality is at the heart of this effort, an ego-driven process that I describe as "pushing." We are pushing when we do battle with the world by attempting to assert our control or mastery over it. We are pushing when we act intentionally to reach the goals we have set or strive to demonstrate our competence as human beings.

Success in these endeavors can be measured by fame or money, but most of the time, success is the satisfaction that comes from functioning in a way that gives us a degree of control. Drive, ego, energy, and effort go hand-in-hand as part of the pushing dynamic. You can make something happen by putting your will and best effort forward behind your intentions. Physical examples of pushing are common in sports, war, and emergency settings, where a burst of energy or heroics determines the outcome.

The Alzheimer's journey is not about ego, however. It's a journey of heart and spirit. Ego quickly becomes a difficult companion. If you continue to push to be part of ego-oriented Earth-reality, you will only add frustration to your journey and diminish the potential for joyful moments. When you break an arm, you wear a cast. When you have chemotherapy treatment for cancer, you lose your hair. When you have dementia, your behavior becomes a bit wacky and unpredictable from the perspective of Earth-reality. You forget things. You don't always do what was expected or respond as quickly and clearly as you did before. The meaning of your communications may not always be clear. It's much healthier to laugh at these limitations than fight them. Your friends and caregivers can be of great help here.

Let Your Feelings Guide You

What you are feeling at any moment offers a guide to help you find the source of the conflict between your ego and your heart. Often this conflict is based on the differences between what you are experiencing in your conscious and unconscious minds. Any experience of feelings is really an attempt to bring an unconscious message into the conscious mind.

The source of much frustration, for example, is that what you know and understand unconsciously to be true is inconsistent with what you are experiencing in the world. For instance, you know you are still an adult, not a child, yet the world may want to characterize your behavior as childish. You know what you're attempting to communicate, yet others will often not understand or even listen. Finally, you know in your core mind that you are still present and a complete person, yet what is happening in the shared, conscious world with family or friends may contradict this because you are functioning, as you must, like any person with dementia.

My previous book, *The Long Moment: Communicating with the Alzheimer's Mind*, discusses the differences between the conscious and unconscious experience of Alzheimer's. I make the point that part of what we consider to be our "unconscious" mind is actually the holistic, nonverbal, knowing part of our conscious mind. When you talk to yourself, it is this right-brain part of your mind that is listening. Right-brain consciousness is much less affected by dementia because of its holistic character and the biological fact that the memories it contains are much more distributed throughout the brain than speech-based memories.

For you, living with Alzheimer's, getting in touch with your feelings means using these emotions as a guide to learning when to let go versus pushing. The *feeling* is the message that matters. What you are striving for here is the internal harmony that comes when you are at peace with yourself because your conscious and unconscious minds are not in conflict. Letting go of the negative thoughts and emotions that don't serve you is the key to making this happen.

Letting Go of Memory Testing

There is a tendency in the early stages of Alzheimer's for your family and friends to insist on "testing" you to see what you remember and "how well" you can continue to function in this ego-oriented world. When you are tested in this manner, it is difficult not to try to comply, even if the result is unsuccessful (and probably frustrating). Testing and constant evaluation is a normal part of Earth-reality, but not appropriate for those living on Altzair. The Care Partner Rules of the Road and the communication guidelines in the previous chapters gave you some tools to share with your caregivers to help address this issue from their perspective. The faster they can move on and let go of this kind of testing, the happier you will be and the more joyful long moments you will experience.

Letting go is not a negative concept. It doesn't mean quitting or giving up or accepting defeat. Rather, it means embracing who you are at this moment and finding joy in being this person. It means being "in flow" with who you are as a person with Alzheimer's instead of battling the changes that are taking place. It means educating your caregivers so they can join in this flow. I introduced the concept of the planet Altzair to help make more concrete the idea that the Alzheimer's mind lives in a different world. Explaining to others that you are from Altzair is a way of reminding them that, like any visitor from another culture, you are different and follow different rules.

Finally, letting go is not about dementia—it is a very healthy and essential behavior in Earth-reality, where finding the balance between pushing and letting go is crucial to success.

One of the biggest reasons that your family and others may resist letting go and want to test you is because *they don't understand your journey.* They are uncomfortable with the fact that, in part, you do live in a different world now, a world they don't understand, so they try to pull you back to a place where *they* are comfortable, the domain of Earth-reality. Learning how to avoid doing this will not be obvious to them; in fact, many caregivers demonstrate this testing behavior throughout the entire Alzheimer's process! This is the reason that education about coming to your world and the guidelines presented in the Rules of the Road are so vital to your happiness.

You may want to test yourself at times, just to see if you can still function in Earth-reality. This is OK and normal. Letting go means, however, that you don't judge or evaluate yourself negatively after these tests. Let's face it: You are going to behave at times like an absent-minded professor (me) and seem a bit nutty! That's fine. Everyone from Altzair is like this. Learn to live with it, laugh at it, and not let it interfere with enjoying many meaningful long moments.

When Mistakes Don't Matter

A natural consequence of making mistakes—forgetting things, behaving in unpredictable ways, needing special assistance—is that the world begins to beat you up about it. Even the kindest of caregivers will unintentionally at times communicate their frustrations with you (and others in the world are not nearly as considerate). As a result, you may feel the need to withdraw from the world, to curl up in a ball, and let go of many social interactions just to avoid another failure.

This tendency to withdraw becomes even stronger as the disease advances because your mistakes (from the perspective of Earth-reality) will only increase. Retreating inside yourself offers safety and security—and a temporary hiatus from the continuous challenges this reality presents.

Imagine, for a moment, a world called Dementia Land where your mistakes are the norm and not a thing to be judged, corrected, or even be the basis for assistance unless it was vital for your safety. What would that be like? I think the answer is obvious. You would be much more social and less withdrawn. Alzheimer's is a lonely journey and companionship is greatly appreciated, unless it serves to remind you of your failures. Could such a world every exist? Yes, it could. As you'll learn in Chapter 23, it's located just outside Amsterdam.

The Alzheimer's Café, skilled caregivers who "come to you," the nuns who lived with Alzheimer's without showing the typical symptoms—all of these are situations where you, the person with dementia, are completely accepted. There is much to be learned here.

Humor is a Key Part of Letting Go

Learning to laugh at your mistakes is essential to letting go. You will make mistakes. Expect them to happen. Embrace them, accept them when they do occur, and, if possible, find humor in the situation—or at least don't take it too seriously. One class I offered for many years at TCU was called "Failure Training." Yes, I actually had my students do projects where they were bound to fail. Does this sound crazy? I had two clear objectives. First, to help them learn to get over a fear of failing, by creating an environment where failing was the norm. Second, to demonstrate to them that in "failing," you often can find your biggest successes. If you have Alzheimer's, you are going to have some failures. No big deal. They won't prevent you from living a full and joyful life unless you let them. Here are some brief reminders to help with letting go.

- Remember that you live on the planet Altzair. It is expected that you will appear to be a bit out of step with people in Earth-reality.

- There is no evaluation on Altzair, only acceptance. Relax and smile at your mistakes.

- You don't need to be out there battling to be competent in Earth-reality terms. Savor your long moments and let your caregivers and friends come to you.

- You will be frustrated at times; that comes with the territory. When you feel frustrated about something, picture it in your mind, take a deep breath, and release it.

- Slow down and allow those around you to give you help and support. Train them to be patient with you.

- Think of your journey with Alzheimer's like a special cruise through your world of family, friends, places, and things that you know, but remember that you are now a passenger on this trip, not the driver.

One of the most significant changes in your experience of the world may be connected with your perception of time: the future, past, and present. A big part of letting go is learning to accept and flow with these changes instead of battling them. The next chapter addresses this important topic.

KEY POINTS

- Your behavior in Earth-reality is often guided by a complex set of social norms or rules and it is judged based on how well you do.

- Much of this behavior is ego-oriented and connected with our need to be competent, successful, and appreciated in this world. I describe this behavior as *pushing* when we do battle with the world in attempting to assert our control over it.

- The concept of *letting go* means to release the need to control, manage, and judge what is happening in the world around you—instead, simply observe it and join it in flow.

- Your journey with dementia is not about pushing or controlling or ego. It is a journey anchored in heart and spirit and feelings. To make this journey and live fully and happily, it is essential to let go of your old, ego-oriented way of living.

- How you feel is an excellent guide for deciding when you can listen to your ego versus when you need to let go. Negative feelings are often a signal that it is time to step back and let go.

- Letting go is not about quitting. It means embracing who you are at the moment and finding joy in being this person.

- Making mistakes is a part of both Earth-reality and living with dementia. The difference is that in Dementia Land, we choose not to judge a mistake. Instead, we accept it and learn from it.

- Humor is your ally in letting go. Your behavior with dementia may be a bit odd. Your life will be happier when you learn to view it lightly and humorously instead of judging or evaluating.

Ideas for your life? How might you act on them? What is the first step?

20

Living with the Changes in Your Perception of Time

I guess not having the ability to look at the past makes it easier to look at the here and now. The past is what we had, the present is what we have now and the future, well, there's no certainty as to what we will have.
—Brian LeBlanc, from his blog, *Alzheimer's: The Journey*

The dimension of time is another part of your reality that, today, is taken for granted. The short-term memory loss associated with Alzheimer's will disrupt things; changes will occur in your perception of time. You cannot prevent these changes from occurring, but you can prepare for them. This chapter briefly outlines what you can expect and how a combination of caregiver education, technology, and your own preparations can help.

Currently, you experience time as a three-dimensional concept. At any moment in your mind, you can be experiencing the present, referring back to the past for guidance, and looking forward to the future to consider the results of your actions. Playing football, for example, draws on a rich past history of well-rehearsed physical skills, experience in similar situations, knowledge of players and teams, and much more—all brought into the present by your mind to help you execute a play. It is also possible in that moment (although not typically helpful) to think forward to the end of the game, to victory, the bus ride home, or perhaps a late date. It is comfortable and normal for all three dimensions to be in play at any moment in time.

This familiar way of perceiving the world is about to change for you. Most people with Alzheimer's will experience a gradual shift in time from three dimensions to a single dimension—the present. The past and future will largely vanish from your consciousness as your mind focuses more and more on what is occurring now. Why does this happen?

To a large degree, it is because the past and the future are concepts created by our mind, not concrete, real things that are part of our experience in the moment. We always live in the present tense even though we are aware of our past and future, but these latter concepts are actually abstractions that we learn to use to influence the present. For example, looking backward, joyful memories from previous holidays can make today's holiday experience even more special. On other hand, looking forward to a desired future can direct our behaviors positively in the present or generate negative emotions based on concerns over a perceived outcome. Alzheimer's brings you back to a single dimension of time, that part that is real and happening now, not what is imagined.

How do you prepare for and then deal with the changes that will take place in your perception of time? I have four suggestions for you, all based on the idea that our experience of time is divided into brief intervals or moments that can range from a few seconds to a few minutes to an hour. In *The Long Moment: Communicating with the Alzheimer's Mind*, I recommended using the "long moment" as the unit of time. By focusing at this level, we have a window into what you are experiencing. Living your life to its fullest with Alzheimer's has many dimensions, but ultimately it reduces to a single common theme—adding positive, quality moments in the present tense.

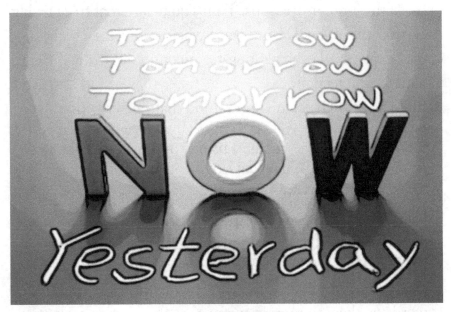

Managing the Changes

You can manage the changes in your perception of time in ways that support living a full and complete life by doing the following.

1. Accept the shift from three time dimensions to one gracefully.

Trying to recover the past dimension is similar to trying to recover lost memories with Alzheimer's. It's not going to happen. The harder you try, the more you are memory-testing yourself, which can be very counterproductive. It's fine to remember the concept of the past and, at times, memories and experiences from the past. But, as you know from Chapter 19, you cannot push here. Letting go of the need to travel back along the past dimension at will, especially the short-term past, is simply part of your journey.

Connecting with the past and your history is still important and healthy for many reasons. That's quite different from trying to recover the immediate past and what occurred an hour, day, or week ago. To keep the long-term connections alive, I have several recommendations:

- Build and use the companion mind that I described in Chapter 12. It sets you up to take advantage of the powerful set of tools for accessing and using your personal history that will come with new developments in technology.

- Rely on the personal anchors described in Chapter 11 to help blend your history with the present. Knowing you are a grandfather or musician or Sierra Club member can change your interactions with family and friends in the present.

- Create a set of Reminisce Cards and use the pictures and words on them to prompt memories. These cards are available on my website at MindPartner.org.

- Encourage your family and caregivers to stimulate your memory by gently leading you down a path that leads back to your life history. Ask them to do this is in a manner that doesn't test you but simply allows you to share a caregiver's recollection. A caregiver might say, "I'm remembering some of the things we did on our vacations. I love the beaches at Hilton Head and the sound of the ocean. You love swimming in the ocean." In this way, you can enjoy your history without feeling pressured.

2. Accept the moment or "long moment" as the unit of time that matters in your experience.

I've recommended throughout the book that you focus on living quality long moments. Now you understand why. Alzheimer's forces you to live in the moment and quality time in your life is measured by the number of good moments that you experience. All of your experiences in a typical day are made of long moments. Focus on these and let go of the past and future.

3. Take the power from negative moments by replacing, not ruminating on, them.

You know that the happiness, joy, and other positive feelings you experience each day depend on the quality of the long moments you are living. Any moment that is grounded in anxiety, stress, unhappiness, frustration, or any other negative emotion is not likely to be a positive one. It would be convenient to simply push away these negative moments in your mind when they occur but, as you know, this is not easy or practical to do. Instead, get rid of them by replacing them with something neutral or positive. Every chapter in this book offers suggestions to help you do this.

A negative feeling is really a signal that something is not right. Often this represents a conflict between your conscious and unconscious minds. Your ego is not in charge now, so let go of the conflict and negativity. Find some new thought or activity to bring you back to the present moment.

Let's look at a concrete example. You're probably feeling some stress or unhappiness associated with your Alzheimer's diagnosis. This condition is likely to persist, because it's not easy to banish. Willing it away simply won't work, but replacing these thoughts with a hobby, a conversation, a game, a meal, a walk, or any number of other positive, concrete things will help—in the moment.

Set Up Positive Moments Using the Power of Precognition

This fancy term from cognitive research simply means that what you are experiencing now was "primed," or set up by previous events. If a person frowns at you before they speak, it's natural for you to expect them to say something negative. A smile produces the opposite expectation. You and your care-givers can help set up the opportunity to experience positive moment by doing the following:

• Using positive, encouraging facial expressions

• Displaying positive, welcoming body language

• Listening carefully

• Selecting warm, empathetic words and phrases

• Remembering these guides: No questions; no criticism; no contradictions

• Being fully present in the moment

The affirmations described in Chapter 16 are one positive form of priming. Think of priming as tuning the stations on your radio. When you tune into happy, positive thoughts, you interpret what you are experiencing now in a positive manner. Negative stations have the opposite effect.

In Earth-reality, I can often separate the precognition or priming influence from the actual event in time and deal with both. On Altzair, for you, these two things are confounded. You may not be able to overcome the weight of the negative first impression and deal with the actual event that you're expe-riencing in a positive manner. Even though you will be living in the "now," what you are experiencing is still strongly influ-enced by unconscious events that prime this experience. The communication guidelines in Chapter 18 are also an excellent reference for your caregivers to support positive priming.

Embrace Repetition or Recycling When It Occurs

The key unit of time in your mind will become a "long moment" or chunk of time tied to a specific experience. In your reality, your experience of an hour, a day, or a week of time will often not match that of your caregivers and friends. Normally, your short-term memory would provide a bridge that allows all of the long moments in a day to be processed, stored, and retrieved later. Without this bridge to help you remember and prevent repetitions, you can relive the same moment many times without being aware that this is happening. Within your own mind, this process of recycling will be normal and not stressful, because there will be no history of previous, similar moments. Under no circumstances is it appropriate for your caregivers to attempt to pull you back to Earth-reality by pointing out the repetitions. Their job is to support you and let go of their own needs to bring you back to their world.

Pattern or repetitive behavior is a normal part of the Alzheimer's process. It is very helpful to think about a repetitive moment as one in which at the beginning of each new cycle, you are waking up to a new day. I am very optimistic about the potential of new technology to help with this waking up process by supporting you in a positive way and by giving your caregivers special tools to help. As your mind repeats a pattern, think of a glide path that gently returns you to the present moment in a healthy and harmonious way.

Your experience of time may change, but your potential to enjoy many positive long moments in the "now" will remain largely intact. Essential to enjoying these moments is accepting yourself, as you are now, with a certain lightness of being and in good humor. The next chapter describes some ways you and your caregivers can add joy by embracing the comedy and humor in your life with dementia.

KEY POINTS

- Alzheimer's and other forms of dementia may shift your perception of time from a continuum with three dimensions (past, present, and future) to one dimension (the present).

- Even though in Earth-reality we live only in the present tense, we are able to imagine the concepts of a past and future tense and use these as part of our experience.

- The key unit of time while living with dementia is the "long moment," or a brief period ranging in most cases from a few minutes to an hour. During this period, you are able to keep your attention focused on one subject or activity without losing track.

- Living a full life with Alzheimer's means adding as many positive, quality long moments to your everyday experience as possible—in the present.

Here are five suggestions for accomplishing this:

1. Accept the shift from three time dimensions to one gracefully.

2. Recognize that the "long moment" is the unit of time that matters in your experience. Life is really just a sequence of long moments.

3. Take the power from negative moments by replacing them with neutral or positive ones, not ruminating on them.

4. Use the power of affirmations to tune your mind to receive positive versus negative signals from the world.

5. Embrace repetition or recycling if this occurs. In your world, each new cycle is similar to waking up to a new day.

Ideas for your life? How might you act on them? What is the first step?

21

Finding Relief in Comedy and Humor

Certainly Alzheimer's is an awful disease, and there is nothing funny about it. But there are funny moments that happen. When you laugh, you're not laughing at them; you're laughing because the moment is funny.
—Cindy Laverty
"The Lighter Side of Caregiving: Appreciate the Humor," AgingCare.com

An important part of living with Alzheimer's or any form of dementia is being able to poke fun at yourself or your behavior. Accepting your "oddness" and finding a way to laugh about it at times is very healthy. Humor allows you to step back from the frustration you might feel as you see yourself behaving in an unusual manner and to move to a place where the behavior, like a cast on your broken arm, is just another part of your reality, not you.

Humor offers other priceless benefits in your social interactions with caregivers and others. Because they cannot see into your mind and consciousness to understand what you are thinking and feeling, they may be inhibited in their interactions with you. They can want to pull you back into speech-oriented Earth-reality and may struggle when they see this is not working. Humor cuts through this noise like a laser in the dark. It offers an immediate, common denominator for communications that you can both share. It can defuse the tension between you in an instant.

Your appreciation of humor will stay with you, in some form, throughout the Alzheimer's journey. Because the core parts of your mind will always retain knowledge of key human concepts (love, joy, children, birth, death, marriage, sex, hero, villain, and so forth), laughter offers an open communication channel that bridges the gap between the planet Altzair and everyday Earth-reality.

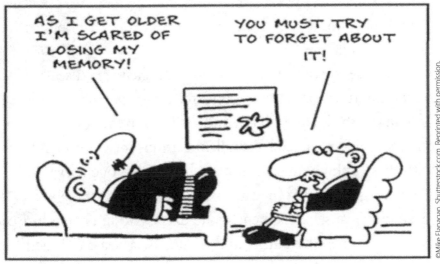

Humor creates the opportunity for conversations that are not about you, which can be very refreshing! Funny stories can make communications flow. And don't forget sex. At times, in an appropriate context, sexy humor, sexy stories, dirty jokes, or any form of communication about sex may be something you will appreciate. Why? Because this is adult talk. Dementia doesn't make you less of an adult, but adult humor is likely to be in short supply.

Are They Laughing with You or at You?

Unless you have a mighty thick skin, you will probably not enjoy all the "humor" that comes your way. Humor has many benefits, yet careless attempts at humor by those who are not part of your family can also be painful and inconsiderate. Because dementia has symptoms that are commonly experienced by most non-dementia people occasionally (brief memory loss; responding slowly; acting confused, foggy, or uncertain for a moment), we often associate them with Alzheimer's in a light way that may not be appropriate. We jokingly say, "Bob buttoned his shirt wrong this morning. I guess he is getting Alzheimer's," or "You woke up in a fog today. I hope it isn't early dementia."

Of course, there is no mild form of Alzheimer's disease. The symptoms described above don't reflect your true experience of living with the disease any more than a bump on your skin reflects a hidden cancer. I think the annoyance you might feel with these unknowing attempts at humor (no one is ever going to get it right about your true experience) is something you can live with because of the benefits here. A cartoon or tee shirt or joke or comment by family and friends is, at least indirectly, a look in the eye. Instead of your handicap being ignored, it is being acknowledged. The truth is that you are behaving oddly at times and even if a cartoon only reflects what is happening on the surface here, that's OK. It's the norm. Seldom will others ever get much closer to your true life on Altzair.

Encourage those around you to be bold about bringing humor into your life. Who are you to be offended by anything at this point versus receiving attention that is real and that embraces at least a part of your world? Your caregivers will, I am certain, remember to laugh with you—with love and compassion.

Richard Taylor's voice is very loud and clear here:

For today I'd like to suggest that you use your power of humor to laugh at yourself. Laughter is one of the best forms of natural meditation. It improves the immune system, lowers blood pressure, and diminishes the effects of stress.

A big part of living a complete and joyful life is engaging the world with a light touch and not taking your mistakes or your behavior too seriously. The language of humor is one of the best tools for accomplishing this. Surround yourself with humor. Let your caregivers know how much you appreciate humor. Many books, programs, and apps for seniors today offer cartoons, stories, and humorous facts that you may enjoy.

Finally, your sense of humor and your appreciation for humorous stories or cartoons send a very important message to your caregivers. It reminds them that despite your limitations, you are still here as a conscious, aware, functioning adult. It reminds them of the integrity of your personhood despite living with dementia. And it reminds them that they too are part of the comedy. Their own situations and behaviors can be just as humorous as yours.

KEY POINTS

- Humor plays an important role in living a full life with dementia and Alzheimer's. It allows you to take a step back from the frustrations of the moment and find relief in the comedy of your life and the lives of those around you.

- Your appreciation of humor will stay with you throughout most of your journey with Alzheimer's. It is an open channel that can bridge the gap between Earth-reality and the planet Altzair.

- Humor offers a common understanding of the world that you and your care partners can share and that often cuts through the noise created by communication problems.

- Having a bit of a thick skin can help here, because not all humor directed your way will be timely or appropriate. Because humor is so natural and so valuable, it is better not to be offended.

- Let your caregivers know how much their attempts at humor are appreciated. Tell them what kinds of humor you enjoy the most.

- It's OK to laugh at yourself. Living a joyful life with dementia means accepting your mistakes and imperfections as a natural part of the process.

Ideas for your life? How might you act on them? What is the first step?

EMBRACING TECHNOLOGY TO ADD QUALITY TO YOUR LIFE

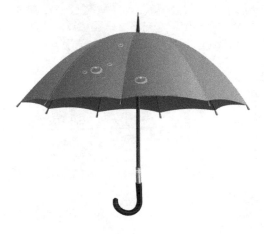

22

Technology and Dementia: Today and Tomorrow

People need to start thinking in terms of how can we enable those living with dementia to function better. How to help them help themselves instead of just taking over everything. How can we enable people to stay at home? Why aren't we using more of the available technology to enable people with dementia to be more independent? Why don't we make things so they DO work for someone with dementia instead of saying they can't do this or that so we have to make sure they don't have the opportunity. We need to start treating people with dementia more like others with different disabilities instead of people who are somehow mentally ill and completely incompetent. If someone loses the ability to walk there are tremendous resources to overcome that disability and continual innovation to make it better. Do you see the same thing happening with the millions upon millions of people with dementia?

—John Sandblom,
Early (Young) Onset Atypical Alzheimer's Disease Blog

This chapter and the next—on creating smart, supportive environments for people with dementia—are more about the future than today, even though most of the technology I describe is already developed. The problem is that it has been created for teenagers, the military, or business—not you. The good news is that this disappointing situation is changing quickly as Apple, Amazon, Google, Samsung, and other major companies, as well as dozens of startups, are creating products to support seniors and in many cases people with dementia. The bad news is that many of these developments offer only limited help because they were created by the technical community, not people living in your shoes. There are a number of dementia-focused apps for mobile phones, for example, yet research suggests that only a small proportion of seniors today are comfortable with this technology.

Can you guess the biggest technical challenge facing many seniors today? No, it is not using their iPhones or computers or elaborate monitoring devices; it is mastering the remote control for the TV! It is no surprise to you that tiny screens, tiny keyboards, and obscure terms derived from an environment managed by programmers are not age-friendly or dementia-friendly.

Looking back a few decades, we can see that the personal computer first gained popularity as a device for playing simple games, creating documents, and doing accounting or other mathematics that replaced the calculator. Then, with e-mail and the Internet, it exploded into communications and the thousands of other applications that we see today. Given the breadth of the developments here, it's actually surprising to me that we don't already have more applications and tools that could benefit you, living with dementia.

Despite these limitations, short of a cure for Alzheimer's, technology represents a powerful ally in support of your goal to live a full life. For you, at this moment in time as you begin your Alzheimer's journey, embracing today's technology may offer the quickest and highest potential path for living independently in the future. Most likely, you are not currently an experienced user of much that current smart, mobile devices offer, such as voice recognition systems, interactive TVs, webcams, video conference tools, virtual realities, and others. That's fine. Fortunately, many of these devices and the services they provide are already being redesigned to work with older populations. Even if you're not familiar with them, you almost certainly have a caregiver, friend, grandchild, or other supporter who is an expert.

Adding technology today to your life is one of the best investments you can make to live fully and joyfully in the future. What does this mean in practical terms? What options should you be considering here now and for the future? Let me suggest an overall vision and then list some areas and tools that might help.

A Vision for Technology in Your Future

The vision I propose comes back to the theme of this book. What can we do with today's technology that will improve the quality of your life with Alzheimer's throughout the entire journey? These improvements must cover many dimensions: maintaining your independence and personhood, supporting communication, adding positive moments and joyful living, aiding your caregivers, making environments friendlier, and so forth. How do we do this? Let's start with a short list of requirements for the best technology-based products. They must:

Listen. They are based on listening to your special needs and requirements first and, to a lesser degree, those of your caregivers, physicians, and facilities.

Target. They must address a specific problem or objective. The concept of an "app" is not very helpful; it is the *service* provided by the app that matters and must be the focus.

Be holistic. They must take a holistic view of dementia and support you within this holistic context.

Be redundant. The best tools will operate like your mind and function redundantly, complementing other tools, lifestyle approaches, or things caregivers are doing.

Fit seamlessly into your life. The tools that you use will be the ones that operate simply and naturally within your world rather than forcing you to do battle with the logic of Earth-reality to master them (which is a major problem with most mobile devices today).

In the next two sections, I will describe: 1) some of the devices that will be used to deliver technology to you; and 2) the services or functions that technology can provide to help you live a full life. Before I begin, however, I want you to ask your care partner to join you for a minute and together read my Dementia Technology Manifesto below. Why? Because current research on dementia caregivers reveals one alarming fact. Fewer than 20 percent of care partners are willing to invest today in technology to help you! Some of this skepticism is justified. Many early experiments with technology had only marginal success, and most devices were not well-designed for seniors. That is no longer true. In the next few years, you will have many options for relevant, helpful tools that can add hundreds of joyful moments to your life. Some excellent products listed below are available now, but you will need help. Start now by enlisting your care partner and your caregiver team. You will want some of this technology, I promise. Here is the manifesto.

Using Today's Technology to Live a Full Life with Dementia

1. I choose to embrace today's and tomorrow's technology, wherever applicable, to add joy and quality moments to my life with dementia.

2. I ask my caregiver team to research and understand the available options here today for people with dementia—and to look for new developments— that can support me in maintaining the integrity of my personhood.

3. I understand that my needs for specific kinds of support will change as my dementia progresses and I know that my team will be watching for these changes and providing the technology needed at the moment that is most appropriate.

Thanks to everyone on my team for your support!

Devices Used to Deliver Technology

In the next two sections, I have separated the tools or devices used to *deliver technology to you* from the *services provided by that technology* because a single tool, such as a smartphone, can perform many different functions ranging from communication to serving as a personal assistant. You will also find that some of these tools will be much friendlier for you than others. For example, less than half of the people in the U.S. over 70 use smartphones, but almost 100 percent do use TVs. It is unfortunate, but much of today's technology is delivered on devices that may not work for you because of size, complexity, or an unfriendly digital language. That is OK. Many of these devices will see improvements in the near future as manufacturers create versions more suitable for seniors, but there is help available now. Your job at the moment is find current technology that can help immediately and is both friendly and offers services you need.

A bigger issue is that you and your adult caregivers will not find it easy to use today's technology when it is presented out of context. In many places below, I tout the potential of smart TVs today for communication, care management and other purposes but are you capable of setting up such a TV to join your caregiver network or track a location sensor that you are wearing? Probably not without some help.

A Glossary of Common Devices for Delivering Technology

The Internet. I know, the Internet is not really a "device," but it is such a key part of much technology today that access to the Internet becomes an essential part of using today's technology. Ask your care partners to be sure your home or apartment has a high-speed Internet connection (assuming this is possible).

Smartphones, Tablets, and Other Portable Devices. There are a hundred options for small, mobile, smart devices today that can serve many functions, ranging from communication to entertainment to personal support. They fall into two rough categories, those manufactured by Apple (such as the iPhone, iPad, or Apple Watch) and Android devices developed by other companies. They are roughly equal in size and features so either choice will work fine. You will probably want to own one of these devices to take full advantage of the technology available. If you find these devices too small and complicated, you may want to consider something like the Jitterbug phone, which is much easier to use but offers many smartphone features—or a tablet-sized device that is easier to view and handle.

PCs. Who uses a PC today, you may be thinking? The answer: lots of people over 70. To many, they are more familiar, have much larger screens for viewing, and are easier to interact with than a tiny pad or phone or laptop computer. Companies such as iNL2 also offer very friendly interfaces designed especially for seniors. It may be helpful to have a PC to set up some of the other devices or programs that you will want.

Interactive TVs. These are a hidden gem that is likely to already be present in your home. They have a wireless connection so they can offer a large display of the screen on your computer or mobile device—and many have a built-in camera for communication. They can function as a TV, a video phone, a monitoring system, and much more.

GPS Tools. GPS is shorthand for location-based technology that can track where you, your friends, the rooms in your house, and most anything else is located. To use it, you carry a mobile device such as a smartphone or wear a bracelet, a pendant, or shoes with a special sole so that the system knows your location. Now and in the future, GPS systems will be the heart of much technology that uses this location information in an intelligent way to serve you.

Headsets. These are already widely used by individuals in the mid to late stages of Alzheimer's to listen to music or stories. They can also be valuable for you now because they can help to shut out the auditory distractions from the noisy world around you to help you concentrate and hear more clearly.

Video Cameras. I am referring to the tiny web cams that are part of many smartphones, computers, interactive TVs, and other devices today. A video cam can share an image of you or your world to support communication with a loved one, use facial recognition tools to identify a person who has just entered the room, interpret your behavior, or provide many other services.

Wearables. These are custom items of clothing or accessories created especially for you. They include watches, shoe soles, bracelets, pendants, smart shirts or coats, hats with cameras, and much more. Working with some of the other products listed in this section, they can track your location, help you communicate, assist with daily habits, and perform a variety of other functions.

Robots and Avatars. This is an exciting and fast-developing area that in the next few years is likely to have some impact on the quality of your life. I will describe their potential in more detail below in the section on caregiving, but some current options include Chihira Aico, Pepper, iRobot, Jibot, Mobiserv, Ed the Robot, and others. Success using robots as caregivers has been modest at this point, but that is about to change.

Smart Environments. You may not think of your home or residential facility as a "device," but a smart environment comes very close to this idea. It can track your location, what you are doing, and what your needs are at the moment and then facilitate you getting these things with reminders, walls that display helpful images, rooms that change to accommodate you, walking paths, doors that open automatically, and much more. Chapter 23 covers this topic in more detail.

Services Technology Can Provide to Support a Full Life

In this section, I describe the functions that technology can provide today and tomorrow to help you live a full life. Remember that currently this is a glass that is 10 percent full—but the tap is wide open and I predict that a few years from now, that number will be close to 50 percent.

Communication. The combination of aging plus dementia can interfere with your ability to communicate with others in many ways. Hands-free technology available on any smartphonephone today, coupled with your interactive TV, can be a big help. You simply say "Call Mary" and a few seconds later, you are talking with your daughter Mary while viewing her on the TV screen!

The "repeat" option on Amazon's Echo or other smart devices can replay the last section of a conversation to remind you of what was said. The next generation of AI-based tools will understand what you might want to say based on place, time, people in the room, and the context provided by the conversation.

Even now, you may have noticed there are times when it is difficult to express a complex idea or feeling with words. Simple tools such as the Alzheimer's Communication Cards or the related app can help here by offering a collection of common messages to select from.

Caregiving. The race is on to find better ways to use technology to support caregiving. There is some urgency here, especially in countries like Japan, where the percentage of younger adults is too small to support a rapidly aging population. The use of robots or smart devices that can assist with daily habits, support mobility, provide companionship, and take on many other basic tasks currently provided by human caregivers is coming soon, with experimental versions available in many countries now.

Virtual caregiving using the communication technology, GPS technology, and habit management technology described in other sections will play a big role in your future. That is why having a care partner team now is so important because your primary caregiver will need this support. Products such as Angela Express by Independa (independa.com) offer a turnkey solution for connecting people with their providers and family members using (as I promised) an HD-interactive TV.

Entertainment. In theory, this is one of the most developed areas since a variety of games, educational tools, and other activities are available now for smart mobile devices and computers. A friendly computer or tablet device offers hundreds of ways to add stimulation to your life, exercise your mind, entertain you, excite your emotions, and connect you with things that add joy or humor. A Kindle or tablet computer can be used for reading or listening to audio books.

Yet, in practice, none of these interfaces may work for you and others with dementia. For example, have you ever played a game on a smartphone? Most people over 70 have not. There is still much work to do here for products that fit your requirements. One of the best examples I've seen that works well in residential facilities is a simulated driving game. You have a dashboard, accelerator, and brake, and can "drive" familiar streets to your home, work, or other places.

Personal Assistants. A full-featured personal assistant can answer questions, make phone calls, provide reminders, get support in emergencies, recognize friends, and much more. While this concept evolved largely as a feature on the iPhone (Siri) and Android phones (Cortana), it is quickly being adapted to special populations such as people with dementia by other manufacturers.

An assistant such as Amazon's Echo product may be worth considering here because training and using it while you are in the early stages may offer significant benefits later when you need more support. Using a personal assistant is perhaps a good first step toward having a robot partner since you have a responsive companion with you from the moment you wake in the morning until you retire for the night. It knows where you are located and what you are doing, and can provide multiple kinds of help, especially with everyday tasks. Forget why you walked into the kitchen? Just say, "Why am I in the kitchen?" Need to check on your meds? Ask, "Have I taken my medications today?"

I recommend that you and your care partner team get to work now on investigating personal assistants. You will want to use one to add independence to your life.

Daily Monitoring. This area could be considered part of what a personal assistant might do, but I see many tools being developed here that focus on this one function, so I am listing it separately. Daily monitoring technology depends on building a special kind of schedule that tracks where you are located and what you are doing throughout the day, organizing this information into a sequence of habits or routines and then providing you with feedback and other kinds of help, when needed.

For more limited health or vital signs monitoring, there are many options available today. You have a choice of basic products that can monitor heart rate, blood pressure, or oxygen levels and smart products that can track sleep habits, watch for long periods of inactivity, or measure changes in glucose levels.

Memory Support. Technology to support lost memory functionality, especially short-term memory, is a really big deal for you and others with Alzheimer's. Built into the idea of personal assistants or daily monitoring tools is everyday, short-term memory support tied to your habits or routines. Devices like WindowMirror (windowmirrorinc.com) that can recover a conversation or replay the history of the last few minutes offer very broad, flexible, short-term memory support. I am expecting to see rapid improvement here as developers become more familiar with the experience of living with the dementia. Today's "Disrupt Dementia" movements around the country are a major force in driving better awareness and understanding of your needs.

Technology that brings your living history into the present as part of your interactions with others offers valuable support in many ways. That personal history can influence the quality of your experiences in the moment (regarding you as a professor or father changes the way that others interact with you) and can support your experiential memory. It also helps to shape our understanding of what will bring you joy or be meaningful to you. This is already happening with music, since some products use a list of your favorite songs or stories to prompt what is playing at the moment.

Companion Mind. I developed the MindPartner program (described in Appendix A) based on the simple idea that every person has a rich, complex personal history that anchors their life and provides a context for how they experience the world. By making parts of this history available to you on your journey with Alzheimer's, as needed, using today's technology, Mind-Partner (mindpartner.org) and similar products such as Mind-Mate (mindmate.org) can support your goal of living a full life.

Urgent Help/Safety. Devices, systems, and environments that offer a quick response and aid in the event of an emergency represent perhaps the most developed area of technology for dementia largely because these products are needed for all seniors. These tools can monitor falls, manage wandering behavior, track vital signs, provide critical reminders, and much more. At the moment, most of these systems are not tied to memory-related behavior but in the future, this is certainly likely. When is a breakdown in daily habits significant enough to warrant intervention? What situations in your life today need the protective net that technology might offer with an urgent help signal?

Connecting with Others. Facebook, YouTube, Skype, and other social media provide a rich panorama of people and their experiences. You can stay in touch with family and friends, get in touch with others who are living with dementia, and explore the world.

Technology in Development

What started a few years ago as a trickle of technology-based products for dementia will be a tsunami in the next few years, adding hundreds of new products, some in time to benefit you. Today, a lot of interesting technology *might* at some point be useful for supporting your life with Alzheimer's. GoPro cameras, for example, offer detailed, personal views of the world that can replace the static webcam. Virtual reality devices are in their infancy at the moment, but soon will be widely available. What if these devices offered a bridge between your worldview with dementia and our shared Earth-reality? Finally, social media for caregiving could connect your mind at any moment with the collective minds of a global caregiver team or a group of people similar to you and living with dementia.

KEY POINTS

- It will come as no surprise that the best technology today was created for teenagers and young adults, not you.

- That is a situation that I and many others are working to change. We believe that today's technology, with mobile phones, smart apps, and smart location tools, can improve the quality of your life with dementia immediately.

- These improvements can cover many dimensions: adding independence, improving your communication skills, helping with everyday habits, and supporting short-term memory loss.

- The best products will:

  1. Listen to your needs (not those of your caregivers).

  2. Target specific problems they can help you resolve.

  3. Be holistic and focused on adding quality to your life now.

  4. Add redundancy by complementing other approaches.

  5. Integrate seamlessly into your life.

- You can begin now by experimenting with social media such as Facebook, using existing devices designed for safety (such as location tracking tools), a mobile phone, tools for entertainment such as a smart TV, health monitors, and emergency devices that provide immediate assistance when needed.

- In the future, it is likely you will have a personal assistant, tools for supporting your daily habits, and cameras that help you see and recognize friends and situations where you might need support.

- Smart environments that "listen" to you will also replace many caregiver functions, making you more independent.

Ideas for your life? How might you act on them? What is the first step?

23

Creating Smart, Supportive Environments

Occasionally, I get lost. I go places I didn't intend to go. I have moments, especially in strange places, when my confusion shifts into bewilderment and I am for the briefest of moments not sure of what is going on around me. It is very difficult for me to accept the idea that I would ever need Safe Return (a nationwide location monitoring system to assist people who become lost) most especially now or tomorrow, or tomorrow's tomorrow.
— Richard Taylor, *Alzheimer's from the Inside Out*

Alzheimer's and most forms of dementia are diseases that typically come late in life. You, of course, already know this since most likely you are in your 70s, 80s, or 90s. Practically speaking, creating an environment that best supports you and enhances the quality of your life has much to do with designs that consider the requirements of both aging *and* dementia. Residential care facilities have made some progress here with designs for aging individuals, but progress to support your needs living with dementia is limited. Having the best dementia-friendly environment for your future, one that is friendly and supportive of your independence, whether it be at a home or residential facility, will depend largely on the decisions you and your caregivers make now.

We all know how frustrating it can be to discover that small things we depend on in our world aren't working. I am, for example, forever misplacing my glasses and then, when the phone rings, searching for them to identify the caller. Today, many of the everyday things you do regularly—waking in the morning, dressing, going to the bathroom, dining, finding clothes or books or other things you need, contacting friends, watching TV, or engaging in activities you enjoy—all take place in an environment where you probably need very little support. This won't be true indefinitely. In the future, you will appreciate living in a place that is designed around your needs, with navigational aids, friendly furniture design, communication aids, and much more.

This chapter describes the concept of an active or "living" environment designed specifically for individuals like yourself, with dementia. It also presents some of the technology needed to make this environment function successfully and make good economic sense.

The really good news here is that our digital technology today has taken our ability to control and manage home environments to a whole new level. While use of this technology to support you or others living with dementia is limited at the moment, that is quickly changing. As this book goes to press, I am working with Roy Montibon and his team to design a new, state-of-the-art facility in Las Vegas, New Mexico, that will incorporate many of the concepts described below for creating a living environment—but what does this mean practically?

A Living Environment

Current homes or other kinds of living facilities tend to be like a lump of rock. They are static and familiar, which is good. Nobody wants a toilet seat that morphs into a pair of hands when you sit. Static environments are passive environments, however. They can't track where you are, what you are doing, and what you need. Their helpfulness is limited to the quality of a design for furniture or equipment that is probably not constructed with your needs today in mind, and other static components such as signs or equipment.

Living environments are interactive environments that take advantage of today's technology to assist you in many ways. In developing the concept of a companion mind, I have assumed that its stored information about you could be used by a responsive, living environment that brings additional intelligence into play when it is needed to help. Living with Alzheimer's means that you will need more help at certain times. Living life to its fullest will depend on having this help.

The key thing that you and your caregivers need to do, right now, is to begin to construct this supportive environment at your home or wherever you are living. You don't have to do this all at once. Most components that I will describe can be added as you need them. But it's important to get started while you are still healthy and can express your ideas about what is needed and how it might be used. Some important components in your living environment will include:

Interactive TV

This is actually a device that you may already have. An interactive TV is simply a normal, flat-screen TV with wireless capability so it can connect with the Internet (part of most TVs for many years) and a web camera. This basic setup allows you to use the TV screen to see and communicate with others and much, much more. Many kinds of intelligence—games, messages, assistance, habit monitoring, for example—can be delivered using this framework. The interactive TV is also how the companion mind described in Chapter 12 will at times communicate with you—and you will communicate with your caregivers.

Recommendation: Add an interactive TV to the room or rooms where you spend the most time.

GPS Tools and Mobile Devices

GPS is short for Global Positioning System, the location-based technology tied to satellites that uses a device like a smartphone or wrist bracelet to identify where you are relative to other things or people in your environment. I described the Samsung app earlier for helping you identify when family or friends are nearby. Your own location can also provide valuable clues for the kinds of support you may need and help keep you from getting lost. Technology is exploding here. In the next few years, you will see many more location-based tools developed to provide assistance. Watches, bracelets, shoes, hats, pendants, and other accessories connected to local GPS devices are already available.

A new generation of products such as iBeacon that use small, local devices instead of satellites to measure your position are now available and will play a major role in supporting location products for homes and residential facilities. In addition to just knowing where you are located, a mobile device can use this location data to guide you with verbal instructions, predict what you are attempting to do, understand what you are saying, and much, much more.

Recommendation: Get a smartphone, tablet, watch, or other wearable with a GPS sensor that you can keep in your pocket or on your body, even if you don't use it immediately. It has the location tools built in that you will need at a later time. Connect to your caregiver team using apps that can support communication and daily activities where you need help. At some point in the future, a lapel camera will also be very helpful to own.

Caregiver Reminders

You're not the only person who can benefit from a well-designed environment. Your caregivers will appreciate an environment with reminders that support their role in assisting you with daily habits, communication, memory support, entertainment, and other areas. You cannot take for granted that they will remember all of the details that come with dementia care, such as the Caregivers' Rules of the Road (see page xvii) or the Communication Guidelines in Chapter 18. Notes and checklists can be a big help. It's not uncommon for caregivers to wonder "What do I do now?" in many situations, or for there to be friends or family who could use some guidance. Richard Taylor offers us a sample list to help with communication from his blog:

Place this on the bathroom door in my room:

Please don't bother asking me what day it is, who is the president. I need to live in and understand what has, is and will happen to me (emphasis on what is happening).

Ask me to repeat what you just told me.

Always introduce yourself and explain why you are here and what you are going to do to me. Pretend I'm your favorite Grandfather.

Ask me about family in the room, my grandchildren, my friends and hobbies, what I accomplished today. What I will do tomorrow.

Please, please help me stay/understand this moment and today.

Orientation Aids

These are simple reminders such as signs on the doors of each room describing its function. Another example, commonly used in airports and public buildings, is arrows on the floor or color-coded walkways that send people in specific directions. A personal assistant on a device like Echo or your smartphone coupled with a GPS device can provide real-time help by guiding you with speech similar to the navigational systems in many automobiles. Not everyone with dementia has difficulty with orientation, but it is common, so be prepared.

Recommendation: Add signs above the entrance to each room identifying its purpose or reminders for things you might be doing in each room.

Mirrors

In Earth-reality, you carry with you awareness of yourself and your location at all times. With dementia, however, it is easy to become disoriented and to lose your sense of where you are, why you are there, and where you were headed. This can lead to wandering or getting lost. Mirrors, especially when placed near doors or other points of exit, can help because seeing yourself in a specific place can break up your trance.

We could count on Dad, who suffered from mild dementia, to wander off at times in any public setting. I remember the chaos at the airport in Dallas as I helped Dad through security first, then went back for Mom only to discover, as we emerged a few minutes later, that he was gone! I spent a frantic 45 minutes, with the help of many airport personnel, trying to locate him. One minute before the plane closed the doors, he showed up, waving from a courtesy cart racing to the gate. He had been located just outside a restroom, confused about which direction to take and looking for help.

Habit Reminders

A habit reminder is a simple tool that prompts a specific habit (such as taking your medicine) or details the sequence of steps that are part of a habit, using a cue card or verbal instructions. To support many daily habits in the future, such as dressing, washing, fixing meals, and so forth, you will occasionally need reminders. It's easy to forget where you are in the sequence when the habit involves a number of steps. And where is the best location for these reminders? That's easy. You want them located at the place in the environment where they will have the most value.

Recommendation: Start simple. Select the daily habit where you have the most difficulty remembering the steps, create a cue card to remind you of the steps you need to follow, and place it in the best location.

Advanced Options

There is much to come here. In the next few years, you will see a plethora of options for providing assistance to the elderly using technology tied to a living environment. New digital devices will recognize where you are located, what you are attempting to do, what you need, what you are saying—and provide feedback or other kinds of support accordingly. I am confident that an environment that understands and supports your needs as a person with Alzheimer's will add joy and diminish some of the frustrations that come from living on Altzair. If this all sounds a bit like science fiction to you, it isn't. If you live in the Netherlands, the future is now for a small population when it comes to dementia care.

Dementia Village

The village of Hogewey, on the edge of Amsterdam, is a remarkable elder-care facility designed for people with dementia and Alzheimer's. It has its own town square, gardens, streets, and other facilities, but only one door as part of a security system to keep residents safe. Caretaker staff pose as members of the village, shopkeepers, police, gardeners, or clerks. Cameras help monitor residents 24/7. Research shows that residents fortunate to be part of Hogewey require fewer meds, eat better, live longer, and are happier than people living in traditional facilities.

The houses in Hogewey have designs ranging from the 1950s to the 2000s to help memory-challenged individuals feel at home in familiar surroundings. Family and friends are encouraged to visit. Only individuals with dementia are admitted and, as you would expect, vacancies are rare. The core idea behind the village is to use an environmental approach to reduce both cognitive and behavioral problems associated with dementia. In other words, to use the environment to make significant, concrete improvements in the quality of life.

The difference between a specialized real-world environment versus a clinical environment (typical in most elder-care facilities) is profound when it comes to supporting the quality and richness of everyday experiences for someone living with dementia. While there is much to be learned here to give us perspective on the best models for treating dementia, the high costs of a program like Hogewey make it impractical for most of today's Alzheimer's population.

What can we find here and use in more traditional memory-care facilities? That's the challenge. How far can we go with technology to meet this challenge, in ways that are cost-effective enough to be widely used? We will see.

As you work with your caregivers to plan your current and future environmental requirements, keep the Hogewey model in mind. Look for ways to create some of the benefits within your own lifestyle circumstances. A friendly and supportive environment is an essential part of person-centered care for anyone nearing the end of life. In the next chapter, we will see how this combines with emotional and intellectual attitudes about death to help create a nurturing end-of-life strategy.

To learn more about Hogewey, see this article in *The Atlantic* (atlantic.com), "The Dutch Village Where Everyone Has Dementia."

KEY POINTS

- The best environments for you are likely be ones that support older people because age and dementia are closely related.

- A "living" environment is a smart, adaptive environment designed specifically for people, like you, living with dementia and focused on improving the quality of their lives.

- It is a good idea to begin now to consider your future living environment. Make some of the changes suggested in this chapter. Take this one step at a time but get started quickly. Here are some tools that can help:

  Interactive TV. Most smart TVs have interactive video, connect with the Internet, and can respond to your voice commands.

  Mobile devices with GPS. The future of smart environments will depend on location-based tools that know where you are at every moment and what you want to do.

  Caregiver reminders. Posters with the Care Partner Rules of the Road, your special needs, and how to communicate can help educate all of your caregivers.

  Orientation aids. Signs and directions that help you orient in complex environments can be a big help. Mirrors help you see yourself in a location to support short-term memory.

  Habit reminders: Simple charts or lists in each room help remind you why you are there.

- Dementia Village: Hogewey, an amazing elder-care facility outside Amsterdam, demonstrates how much a well-designed environment can add to the lives of people with dementia.

Ideas for your life? How might you act on them? What is the first step?

DON'T RAIN ON MY PARADE

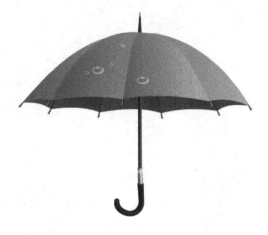

24

Journey's End: Embracing Death

All of this makes me wonder . . . "Do people in the last stages of Alzheimer's still hear and understand but just can't communicate back?" I hope so. I hope I can still hear the voices of my loved ones when my time comes. I want to hear their voices and music and all the things that make me happy. I can only hope.
—Brian LeBlanc, from his blog *Alzheimer's: The Journey*

I can remember writing my eulogy, on a cool, misty spring day, sitting on a cliff overlooking the Pacific Ocean at Esalen, a center for personal growth. Over the years, I would return many times for many kinds of experiences (including two more eulogies). That early lesson on death and life stayed with me in my work as a teacher and psychologist. It also became the core of my new year's planning. If you have only one more year to live, what are the things that you want to be sure are included in your life?

In my work with clients, friends, and family on health-related issues, using guided meditation as a tool to help the mind visualize desired outcomes, I found myself also dealing with the subject of death in cases where the disease was no longer treatable. Then, instead of supporting healing, the conversations often took another course. A common theme was, "Please ask my family for permission to die. I'm suffering now and don't want to hang on any longer for them. I'm ready to go."

These are difficult decisions for family but they are also very difficult for physicians. To them, death, like Alzheimer's disease, represents "losing the war." Atul Gawande makes this point very well in *Being Mortal* where he notes that "[t]he heart of the problem here concerns the function of medicine. We are used to battling death but it doesn't make any sense to be battling for battling sake when there is no chance of winning."

Richard Taylor offers his own thoughts about caregivers for the time when his own death is near:

After they have spent years dealing with the impact of late-stage Alzheimer's on their loved ones I have heard caregivers say out loud, "It would be best for him if he died in his sleep. Mercifully, it should happen sooner rather than later."

Wait a minute here? Can we talk about this before you increase my pain medication? Pull the plug? Withdraw drugs, food or water? What happened to me and the disease being separate entities? Am I now less human? Is my existence diminishing in lockstep and because of the progression of the disease?

As you deal now with your own diagnosis of Alzheimer's, it is difficult to avoid the topic of death. Your death, like the death of your friends and family, is inevitable in time. Death brings finality to something so precious in your life: the living presence of another being on this earth that you love and care for. Contemplating the future death of a loved one or remembering the past death of someone close can take away your breath. It is easy to put off these difficult and emotional conversations. Most people do. Dr. Jenny Randolph, in her research tracking

1,500 families dealing with Alzheimer's over a period of five years, found that fewer than 25 percent had a conversation about death.

This is not a book about death but about living a quality life; however, the inevitability of your death (and mine) serves as a beacon to remind us that time is finite and never long enough. The time to live is now. Your age doesn't matter. At every age, there are moments in the day that offer positive experiences to engage us and feed us joy or interest or comfort. You know that your independence, your social relationships, and your caring for others serve to feed these positive experiences. You also understand that with the help of your caregiver team, and perhaps some changes in your behavior, many additional moments of joy will be available to you.

As part of your long-term planning, I hope that you chose to have "the conversation" about your end-of-life choices with your family members and have created the formal documents needed to support these choices (check back to Chapter 9). If not, stop immediately and make these plans now. In a PBS *Frontline* broadcast, Dr. Angelo Volandes emphatically describes how the current process for advance directives is not working. He notes that rarely was the patient's voice actually preserved when it was needed most—when they could not speak for themselves.

Managing the End of Your Story

As we learned in Chapter 3, an essential part of your story, one that affects the quality of your life and your personhood, is the ending. Your goal here is to end it with comfort and dignity in a manner that you choose. Alzheimer's only complicates this issue because despite what is happening in your mind, you will cross the legally defined threshold of "mental competence" much sooner than people with other diseases. How do you manage your ending now, since you will not have this option later? Here are my recommendations:

1. Join with your family or other caregivers and go to the website www.theconversationproject.org to better understand your end-of-life options. Be sure the options you want are consistent with the advance directives you created in Chapter 9. The most important of these documents is your checklist, which covers all the essential options in very simple, clear language.

2. Next, with your advance directives in hand, take one more step. While a family member videos you (a mobile phone video will be fine), go over the choices and, in your own words, explain what each one means to you. Your expressions and emotions here make it much more likely that physicians and others who see this video later will get things right.

Death is a difficult, emotional topic to discuss in most cultures. As you discuss things that you want to do now, before death, that bring joy to your life (such as the bucket list) or options for where and how you want to end life, a surprising thing happens. Much of the anxiety about death disappears. Instead of a topic to avoid, it becomes a concept that helps you and your family focus on living fully now. Without these conversations, death is always the elephant in the room, lurking in the background with a profound but unspoken presence that can twist emotions or steer family decisions about living now in the wrong directions.

Is there is a compass here that explains how the choices in our lives guide our deaths? Richard Taylor again offers his thoughts:

It is said that most people die the way they lived. If they were generous in life, so too in death. If they were insensitive with their wives and children, so they will approach death in the same manner. I think this is true of my spirit. It evolves as I evolve, and the pronouncement that some disease is gumming up my brain does not in and of itself dramatically influence the possibilities of change for my spirit.

Perhaps the biggest challenge you face in living life to its fullest is keeping the core parts of your current consciousness intact so that you do experience joy and independence, and engage in activities that bring you pleasure and an awareness of who you are and the nature of your journey. I believe that an important part of this process is having access to your personal history through pictures, stories, and videos, and taking advantage of today's and tomorrow's technology as it becomes available.

Finding True North

The Alzheimer's journey is ultimately about spirit. At the moment of your conception, a spark in the darkness of the infinite cosmos was quickly transformed into a living being, you, sailing along the genetic and biological corridors unique to all humans on Earth and joined by spirit. At the end, that spirit—the essence of all that you represent in our living universe and that connects you with all others as one—is alive and well and in communication with those around you. Listen for a moment and inside your mind, you will hear it singing with joy. Ask your caregivers to listen and they too will touch the part of you that is strong and pure and unbroken, despite your difficult travels. Even as they grieve your loss, know that your ending is, in fact, a celebration and your song for them.

Greg O'Brien describes this most eloquently:

While the brain can be dissected, the soul is far more elusive, a place where sparks can miraculously shine through dysfunction.

On the day after Christmas in 1999, I was waiting outside the operating room, working on my laptop, as Mom had surgery for a broken hip. Dad had passed some months earlier and Mom, I knew, was reluctant to enter the next millennium without him. Suddenly, this note appeared on the screen:

Dear Son,

I wanted to tell you that your mother will be leaving you and Nancy and Howard much sooner than you expected. I know you will miss her but she has been very lonely these past months—and is finally coming home to be with me.

I love you son,

Dad

A minute later the door to the operating theater opened and the anesthesiologist, a former student of mine, announced her death, with an expression that spoke of understanding and joy.

KEY POINTS

- If you knew that you would be dying in a few months, what are the things you would like to do now? Writing your obituary is a great tool for reminding ourselves of what we value in life.

- What about conversations that you would like to have with loved ones? Have them now, while you're still healthy.

- The big question, as the story of your life comes to a close, is how to end life with dignity and in a manner you choose. Here are two suggestions:

  1. Go to the website theconversationproject.org to better understand your end-of-life options. Be sure the options you want are consistent with the advance directives you created in Chapter 9.

  2. With your advance directives in hand, take one more step. While a family member videos you (a mobile phone video will be fine), go over the choices and in your own words, explain what each one means to you.

- The Alzheimer's journey begins with words and charts, becomes a matter of heart and feelings, and ends in a place that is ultimately about spirit. Greg O'Brien describes this most eloquently in his book:

  While the brain can be dissected, the soul is far more elusive, a place where sparks can miraculously shine through dysfunction.

- I was present at the deaths of both parents and my son. Their spirits live in me today.

Ideas for your life? How might you act on them? What is the first step?

25

Don't Rain on My Parade

The gift that I want this Christmas is for today, to forget that I have Alzheimer's and for you and others to treat me as you would before the diagnosis. Just for today I want back that life where I am an adult, we can have a normal conversation, you listen to the answers to my questions without wearing your dementia-glasses to filter my responses. When we talk you speak in a normal voice and look me in the eye. There are no conversations between you and others going on around me as if I was not present. Today I am dementia-free.
—Greg O'Brien, *On Pluto: Inside the Mind of Alzheimer's*

This book starts with the premise that each of us was a whole person when we were born, continued to be a whole person throughout our life, and is a whole person now, regardless of whether or not we suffer from Alzheimer's. If you have Alzheimer's, I don't just believe you are "alive" inside the shell of a damaged mind, I believe you are fully alive as an intelligent, emotional being, draped in the rich history of your life experiences, and waiting—hoping and waiting—for the rest of us to break through our fear and negativity and find you.

There is no doubt that the Alzheimer's journey is a difficult one but, as hundreds of stories, blogs, and caregiver reports from families dealing with Alzheimer's tell us, beginning *now*, you have the opportunity of living for years with thousands of quality long moments to look forward to. You know that you create much of your reality with your mind, your intentions, and your choices. In Chapter 1, you made the choice to live life fully and happily. Just making that one decision will have a profound effect on your future life and on your caregivers.

In every chapter, I mention your care partners and how important they are to your health and continued happiness. The primary caregiver's job, even with a full caregiver team behind them, is challenging and time-consuming. All of the team members are required to learn new rules about communication, person-centered care, patience, love, and much more. These are big commitments. You are fortunate to have such a team; however, they are also fortunate to have you. When you made the decision to live completely and joyfully and to let go the negativity that surrounds Alzheimer's, you reciprocated their love for you by caring for them. You opened the door for them to be real partners in your journey. Your experience together is a different experience with your positive outlook, your willingness to plan ahead, and your willingness to focus on the quality of the positive moments you find every day.

This book starts and ends with the integrity of your personhood and your right to live life to its fullest, with or without Alzheimer's disease. It's your parade. No one can end it without your permission. Your compass is your personal well-being, your will to live, your independence, and the joy you experience each day. I hope that you have found some of the ideas in this book to be helpful. You are a true hero on a journey that will take you from comfortable landmarks in our shared reality to another planet. Remember that your essence as a unique person, your core identity, and your spirit will always be with you. My heart goes out to you. Travel well.

APPENDIX A

MindPartner: Apps for People with Dementia

The goal of the MindPartner program (mindpartner.org) is to create a technological toolbox of products to accompany the companion mind that I recommended you create in Chapter 12. Once you have stored your personal history of images, videos, stories, everyday habits, and preferences, what do you do with it? How do you benefit from it? The answer is that you give the intelligence in this "mind" back to yourself through a collection of apps. The term "app" is just shorthand for software or other digital tools that can provide a service for you on any of the devices described in Chapter 22—daily reminders, entertainment, activity or location monitoring, acting as a personal assistant, and much more.

This appendix describes a few of the basic apps I've designed as part of the vision for the MindPartner program. My list is but a small fraction of the set of potential apps currently being developed or that might be developed in the future. Note that some of these apps are already available in MindPartner or products such as MindMate, but others are just ideas at the moment.

Proposed MindPartner Apps

1. **Bucket List.** Create your bucket list, receive daily reminders of your progress in completing the list, and celebrate completed items with fireworks.

2. **Planning.** Find and complete the required documents for healthcare directives, hospice, living alternatives, and end-of-life options.

3. **Communication Cards.** Create a set of cards with pictures and words to communicate things you want to say. Cards can be used directly or delivered via an app on a mobile device.

4. **Reminisce Cards.** Create a set of cards to remember key people, places, and events that are part of your personal history. Cards can be used directly or presented on a mobile device.

5. **Joy Shots.** Build a library of music, pictures, and stories that make you smile, then use it when needed to give you a boost.

6. **Care Partner Team.** Build your caregiver team and then set up schedules and communication tools for working with them directly or remotely.

7. **Comic Relief.** View a library of cartoons and jokes on dementia, aging, and other topics that you can access randomly or by subject on a mobile device or TV.

8. **Habit Sequence Cards.** Build sets of cards to serve as reminders for habits you do each day that involve a sequence of steps, like dressing or preparing a meal.

9. **Environment Cards.** Create cards to serve as reminders of directions, room functions, or places in your environment.

10. **Personhood Anchors.** Create charts to display that remind you of connections with people, organizations, roles, and other personal anchors. These connections can be linked to the Friend Identifier app described below.

11. **Happiness Reminder.** Prompts you to remember things that make you happy to support living positive long moments based on the list you created in Chapter 2.

12. **Avatar.** Select a family member, friend, hero, cartoon, yourself, or any character to serve as a companion for your journey with Alzheimer's. The avatar becomes the "face" of the personal assistant who provides you with apps and other services.

13. **Wake-up Stories.** Create simple cards or videos that are part of a daily timeline designed to support you with a "wake-up story" when your mind loses track of the present and wants to recycle.

14. **Come-to-Me Reminders.** Create signs to post in your home to remind visitors to come to your world with their communications, behaviors, and expectations.

15. **Friend Identifier.** An app, designed for a local GPS network, that tracks your location relative to that of your care partners and other friends. It can announce their presence, remind you of a planned activity, or support your interactions with them by providing cues to prompt a conversation or other details.

16. **My Blog.** A simple "blog" that is set up automatically for you and connects with your care partners and friends. It allows you to share with others anything you want to say about your experience with Alzheimer's.

17. **Adopt a Pet.** Go to the "MindPartner Pet Store" and adopt a digital pet! You can select a pet that is in constant need of your assistance to survive or an independent one that occasionally needs your care and attention.

18. **Frustration Popper.** Choose from a set of cartoons, pictures, or statements to define your favorite frustrations; then enjoy attaching them to a set of digital balloons and popping them to release the tension they create.

APPENDIX B

Online Resources

Dementia Action Alliance USA
www.daanow.org

Alzheimer's Society (UK)
www.alzheimers.org.uk

Alzheimer's Reading Room
www.alzheimersreadingroom.com

Dementia Action Alliance UK
www.dementiaaction.org.uk

Alzheimer's Canada
www.alzheimer.ca

Memory Bridge
www.memorybridge.org

Alzheimer's Australia
www.fightdementia.org.au

Dementia Alliance International
www.dementiaallianceinternational.org

Life Changes Trust (Scotland)
www.lifeschangestrust.org.uk/people-affected-by-dementia

Dementia Mentors
www.dementiamentors.org

Innovations in Dementia (UK)
www.innovationsindementia.org.uk

I'm Still Here Foundation
www.imstillhere.org

Partnerships in Dementia Care Alliance (Canada)
www.uwaterloo.ca/partnerships-in-dementia-care

Dementia Diaries (UK)
www.dementiadiaries.org/uk

The Purple Elephant (Canada)
www.thepurpleelephant.org

Dementia Friends (UK)
www.dementiafriends.org.uk

Teepa Snow
www.teepasnow.com

Mindset Centre for Living with Dementia (Canada)
www.mindsetmemory.com

Murray Alzheimer Research and Education Program (Canada)
www.waterloo.ca/
murray-alzheimer-research-and-education-program

Alzheimer Society of Ireland – Living With Dementia
www.alzheimer.ie/living-with-dementia

Memory Care Café
www.memorycarecafe.org

Memory Café USA Directory
www.memorycafedirectory.com/state-directories

Scottish Dementia Working Group
www.sdwg.org.uk

Dementia Engagement and Empowerment Project (UK)
www.dementiavoices.org.uk

Forget Me Not Online Support Group
www.sites.google.com/site/forgetmenotgroup

Mick Carmody
www.carmodym59.com

Glorious Opportunity
www.gloriousopportunity.org

ARTS & MUSIC

Alzheimer's Poetry Project
www.alzpoetry.com

To Whom I May Concern (theater program)
www.towhomimayconcern.info

Arts4Dementia
www.arts4dementia.org.uk

Dementia & Imagination (arts)
www.dementiaandimagination.org.uk/art-and-dementia

Dementia Arts
www.dementiaarts.com

Meet Me at MoMA
www.moma.org

Creative Dementia Arts Network (England & Wales)
www.creativedementia.org

ACKNOWLEDGMENTS

want to thank the many people who assisted me in some way in the planning and preparation of this book. For encouragement about the idea of creating a positive book on Alzheimer's, I am grateful to Jytte Lokvig, Carolyn Moore, and Ariella Robbins. For reading my early drafts and providing excellent feedback, I want to thank Cindy Lux, Shirley Hirsch, Alan Webber, Roger Taylor, Judy Tuwaletstiwa, Karen Love, and other friends. For helping produce the final manuscript and artwork, I want to thank my editors Sheila Buff and Morgan Farley, my proofing editor Ruth E. Thaler-Carter, my cover and layout designer Peggy Nehmen, and other designers Amiel Gervers and Cindy Lux. For many of the ideas in the book plus stories and quotes, I am indebted to the courageous community of individuals living with dementia and their caregivers who shared their experiences in books and blogs. This group includes Richard Taylor, Greg O'Brien, John Sandblom, Brian LeBlanc, and a dozen others. I was fortunate to meet Brian in my work with the Dementia Action Alliance and am very thankful for his amazing Foreword. For welcoming me into the person-centered care community and reminding me that others have been focusing on living a full life with dementia for many years, I would like to thank Karen Love, Jackie Pinkowitz, Lori La Bey, and other members of my Dementia Action Alliance workgroup. Finally, I would like to think my spouse Marilyn for her patience and support during this planned three-month project that kept changing and expanding until it became a two-year odyssey.

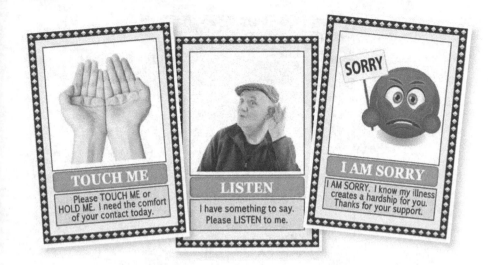

ALZHEIMER'S COMMUNICATION CARDS

The Alzheimer's Communication Cards are tools to help people with dementia communicate with care partners and friends. They are especially valuable when verbal/logical speech processes have deteriorated.

Each card contains an image and a word or sentence that express the message to be communicated. They are divided into eight categories covering issues such as Needs, Feelings, or Things I Want to Say.

Two sets of 72 Alzheimer's Communication Cards are available:

• **Standard Deck:** for people with very limited verbal skills; has simple words and phrases.

• **Advanced Deck:** for people able to use more complex words and expressions in their communications.

Order now at: AlzheimersCards.com or CimarronInternational.org and click on the Products section.

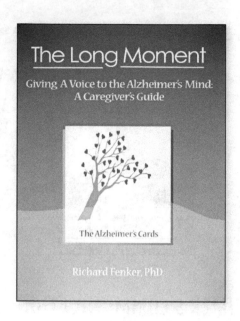

ABOUT THE AUTHOR

Richard Fenker, PhD, is the co-chair of
the Dementia Action Alliance's National
Committee on Technology and Dementia and creator of the Alzheimer's Communication Cards. He is also the inventor of the MindPartner program, which
stores the personal histories of people
with dementia in a "companion mind"
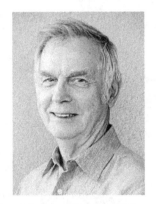
they can use for support. Dr. Fenker is also the author of *The
Long Moment: Giving A Voice to the Alzheimer's Mind.*

Professor emeritus of Psychology at Texas Christian University, he is known internationally for his work in cognition,
sports psychology, and forecasting. A National Science Foundation Fellow, Dr. Fenker was sport psychologist and science
director for the U.S. Gymnastics Team. He is an entrepreneur
and founder of several companies, and was recently honored
as a leading technologist in New Mexico in *Business Weekly's*
"Who's Who in Technology." Dr. Fenker lives with his wife
Marilyn in Santa Fe.

9 780989 460019